TEN GOLDEN RULES FOR GOOD HEALTH

Nature's Best Series

Jan de Vries

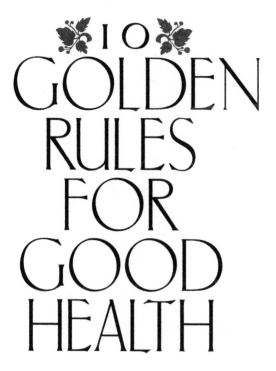

10 GOLDEN RULES FOR GOOD HEALTH

MAINSTREAM
PUBLISHING

EDINBURGH AND LONDON

First published in Great Britain in 2001 by
MAINSTREAM PUBLISHING COMPANY (EDINBURGH) LTD
7 Albany Street
Edinburgh EH1 3UG

ISBN 1 84018 431 0

A catalogue record for this book is available from the British Library

Typeset in Berkeley and Manson
Printed and bound in Great Britain by
Creative Print and Design Wales

contents

Introduction

Often, when people come to see me, I tell them they should try to eat and live healthier. For me it is easy to give such advice, but even if they have read a dozen health books, patients usually do not know how to follow my advice, as most of what is written about health is extremely confusing. Many people understand what is meant by 'a healthier way of living'. They know that they should stop smoking, take more exercise and get more sleep. However, they often do not understand what kind of food they should eat and, above all, they do not know *why* they should eat in such a way. Many serious and also less serious specialists or health food fans recommend all kinds of special diets. It may be all right to follow such a diet for a certain length of time, when people are suffering from some specific ailment, but such a diet cannot possibly be continued for the rest of one's life.

In the back of my mind I always had the idea of writing a book, wherein I would explain *why* 'modern food' is a real, and the most important, cause of our society's diseases. I also wanted to explain why modern food endangers our health in that it cannot be assimilated, processed and used in an optimum way by our bodies.

In this book I will draw your attention to the fact that since the earliest beginnings, the infrastructure of our intestinal tract has been intended for the processing of natural foods. Food that has been artificially altered does not belong in the human body and will sooner or later be harmful to us. I will prove the above statements while looking at them from every possible angle and I hope that after reading this book you will be convinced that we should try to change our eating and living habits. Nobody wants to be chronically ill for the rest of his or her life and everyone is responsible for his or her health.

This is only the first part of the series. There are several more to follow. In this first section, as I have said, I have examined many angles relating to obtaining and maintaining optimum health.

Although I have practised for over 40 years within the field of complementary medicine, I will not claim to know all there is to know on the subject. However, I knew a man who, next to Dr Vogel, knew more than anyone about food and our eating patterns, as well as the dangers of eating certain foods. At the beginning of the Seventies, I attended a conference in Switzerland and, I am sure, due to divine intervention, bumped into a gentleman who was talking to one of my friends, a professor in medicine. I couldn't help but overhear the conversation and, fortunately, my friend introduced me to this special man with whom I would become very friendly. I found his views most interesting and I soon discovered that he was not only very intelligent, but also had a great wealth of experience and knowledge. The man in question was Dr K.O. Heede. He was full of enthusiasm about his work and had a real devotion to his patients. His knowledge was so extensive that I truly regard him as one of the greatest figures of the twentieth century. At the same conference I met a very good friend of his, Marie-Louise Schicht, a very well-known naturopath. It was fortunate that this equally intelligent lady managed to learn and collect Dr Heede's work and, following his death, accumulated a great deal of information on his work. Luckily, some of this knowledge has been shared with me.

I have been most fortunate to meet such wonderful and dedicated people in my lifetime, and I want to present this knowledge to others in order to benefit and improve their health. Therefore, when my publisher asked me to write a book which would be easy to understand, I was delighted to be allowed to use a lot of their work and material. I am confident that this book, which is so special as a result of the contribution of these two people, will be an indispensable and informative guide to those who are seeking better health and a better future in today's society.

To demonstrate the love and interest that Dr Heede had for his fellow beings, he wrote a letter to the British Medical Association on 25 March 1984. The following letter demonstrates the considerable foresight that Dr Heede had regarding ill health and the treatment of disease. In addition, a great deal of Dr Heede's findings and work is included in this book.

In the second volume of this series, I will explain why today the wrong treatment of acute diseases and the suppression of symptoms can be the cause of most chronic diseases. In the third volume I will point to excellent old and new yet little-known healing methods.

Dear Colleagues

To my surprise I have learnt from a German periodical for natural healing methods, that a study group promoted by you will clarify why during the last decades natural healing methods have gained an ever-increasing number of followers and why herbal cures, meditation, the laying on of hands, acupuncture, etc. seem to help people more than medicaments and highly developed technology.

In over 45 years of medical practice, it has become clear to me that the human being is a part of nature and not a chemical laboratory. In case of illness he has the burning desire to be healed. However, healing is a natural process and not a chemical reaction. In spite of these incontestable facts, and although we were taught in school that physics, chemistry and biology are three totally different subjects, which should be kept apart, it seems that in scientifically progressive medicine it is believed, even today, that it is possible to produce chemical reactions in a biological organism and in this way heal a disease.

Each year this so-tragic error costs the lives of millions of people or brings them suffering and chronic invalidism. No wonder that more and more patients are disappointed and turn their backs on scientific medicine in order to be healed by natural methods, or at least improve their poor health. Even the shiny, chromium-plated examining apparatus of a technically perfectly equipped medical practice, X-rays and laboratory tests, cannot fool the patient in the long run, as in this way only the symptoms of a disease can be registered, saying nothing about the cause. However, it will never be possible to heal a disease if the cause cannot be recognised. Only when the cause is known can it then be removed with naturally effective healing methods.

At all times, the foundations of medical science are based on the belief and the assumption that only those things exist and should be scientifically recognised which can be seen, measured and weighed. But it is known that there are more things between heaven and earth than those our school wisdom has taught us and which can be seen with the lifeless eyes of measuring science. However, only the active unseen forces which move this world decide about health and disease, life and death. This is of the utmost importance for successful medical practice and success at the sickbed.

Just as the ability to recognise the cause of a disease from the visible symptoms is indispensable for the right diagnosis, the removal of the cause is also indispensable when healing a patient. The knowledge of the autonomous control regulations in and outside the human organism and the body's self-defence and self-healing forces is at all times the determining factor. The self-healing force of the human body is the only physician in the world who is able to heal a disease. For many people it is an inexplicable mystery why natural therapies like herbal cures, meditation, laying of hands, acupuncture etc. can cure an illness. But hereby the defence and self-healing forces of the organisms are activated, contrary to the registration of symptoms with highly technical instruments and the fight against those symptoms with dangerous chemotherapy.

As we have seen through experience at the sickbed, most now 'incurable' diseases could be cured by activating the body's self-defence and self-healing forces in a comparatively easy way, if the treating physician had learnt how to heal during his studies. Here the most important prerequisite is not to treat the disease, but to remove the cause. It is, for example, not possible to heal bronchial asthma when the patient is being maltreated with the usual chemical anti-asthmatic and bronchospasmolytics. However, when the cause is removed healing is possible and the cause of this problem is always fundamentally a disturbed or abnormal bacterial flora. All diseases of the lymphatic organs, like sinusitis, chronic bronchitis, allergies, rheumatic diseases etc. have the same origin.

It is only possible to treat circulatory problems successfully and prevent a stroke or a cardiac infarction when the cause is eliminated. This means the removal in most cases of the existing protein and cholesterol deposits on or in the walls of the blood vessels (for example by frequent blood-letting) and the treatment of the inflammatory changes in the walls of these vessels with appropriate biological measures.

No migraine or recurrent headache can be cured with the normally used ergotamine, caffeine, or phenacetin containing antalgics etc. However, a cure is very possible with natural therapies and the treatment of the regulatory disorders of the autonomic nervous system and the sympathicotonic reactions.

For more than 2,000 years, experienced physicians have known that most eczemas and skin diseases can be seen as the endeavours of the organism to remove metabolistic residues, toxins etc. by way of the epidermis. They know how to activate these elimination endeavours and thereby heal the disease within a short time. Today, one believes that by chemically suppressive measures and externally applied creams and lotions one is able to remove the problem, of course without lasting success and possibly with the consequence of new and different health defects.

The generally accepted medical dogma that in the case of cancer the symptoms, the tumour, should be removed by operation, after which the patient, who has been weakened by radiation and poisoned by chemotherapy, can be discharged seems almost naïve. If, in spite of the massive application of all technical and other means which we use in the fight against cancer, so far we have had no success, this proves once again that all illness is only curable when the cause, and not the symptoms, are removed. This is valid just as much for cancerous diseases as for other health disturbances.

Just as in all diseases, the symptoms, in this case the tumour, is not just a local symptom which can be removed and destroyed by steel, rays and chemotherapy, from which the patient often perishes, but the consequence of a fundamental impairment of the entire organism. In this connection the development of cancerous cells or the change of normal cells into cancerous cells is always only the consequence of the disturbance, because the real cause for the development of cancer is due to the breakdown of the immunological defence restrictions. Only then is the multiplication of cancer cells possible – never before. However, now, as before, scientific medicine takes the view that only after a radical removal of the tumour, radiation and the necessary chemotherapy treatment can the patient be free of his or her disease. This kind of view not only shows the unwillingness to look for causal correlations but is the prerequisite for the failure of the prevailing and customary treatments of this medical epoch. It could easily be proved by many examples that only a causal treatment, while observing the biological conditions, can give us a chance of success.

Innumerable remedies and natural healing methods are available for the treatment of acute and chronic disease, chiefly in Germany. As long as natural healing methods and remedies are ignored, the consequences are particularly tragic, as millions of people could be cured by them. Now, without biological treatment, these people often suffer painfully for years and die early.

Not only in Europe, but in other countries overseas more and more voices can be heard criticising the use of chemotherapeutic agents. Such remedies might perhaps be needed in case of emergency, but should never be used in the daily treatment of acute or chronic illness. In Germany especially, where natural medicine has been practised and recognised for a long time, many physicians know that this is the only possible way to heal a patient while not risking the danger of side-effects. And because the patients are realising more and more that the suppression of symptoms has nothing to do with the curing of a disease, these biological healing methods are, without doubt, the therapy of the future.

CHAPTER ONE

Nutrition

Let us try in our *Ten Golden Rules for Good Health* to begin with ten rules for healthy eating. I shall try and embroider a little bit upon this, with some back-up from Dr Heede and my colleague Marie-Louise Schicht.

The ten rules for healthy eating are of paramount importance when striving for good health. You may have been learning many different things about the structure of your body and about diseases which have been caused by changes in your nutrition and lifestyle. Now you probably wish to know what you should change in order to successfully prevent the previously mentioned problems, or maybe undo any harm which has already been done. Maybe you skipped the introduction because you were more interested in the practical part. If this is the case it is not necessarily wrong, but it will be more difficult for you to understand some of my recommendations than it would have been if you had read the start of the book. Therefore, perhaps you will be encouraged to catch up on this.

Many diseases and health problems – I hardly have to stress – are not destiny, but the results of our way of living. There are things in life which one cannot, or can only with difficulty, change, such as the condition of our environment. But other things can be quite easily influenced by us. One of these is our nutrition. To deal consciously, and intelligently, with the problem of your eating habits will pay dividends many times over. As you have seen, nutrition not only determines the condition of our digestive systems but also influences in an indirect manner, by way of our blood and lymphatic fluids, all the other organs in our bodies.

Now, what would we call 'a healthy way of eating'? This question has already been raised at the beginning of this book. After looking at the historical background of our development and biological foundations, the answer is easy: healthy food is that which the human being, in the course of his development, has found in his natural environment. His body has adapted to this kind of food and it is easily digestible for him. Modern nutrition in the industrial countries hardly fulfils these requirements. A short-term adjustment of the body to society's new nutritional conditions has been impossible, and the consequences are logical and in accordance with this. If humanity had been able, one million years ago, to eat as we eat today, it is likely that an adequate adaptation might have been possible. The intestines would have become shorter, the pancreas and the liver would have become bigger, and the teeth and the lower jaw would have become smaller.

Now, in order to eat healthily, we should follow as much as possible the example of our ancestors. We should try to eat the food which, over a great many long stretches of human history, has become natural to us. As our 'normal' nutrition, today's way of eating, is much different from the ancient way of eating, the following rules may seem very demanding to you at first. However, this does not mean going without food that you like altogether. Food should and has to taste good! Even when following these ten rules exactly, you can have meals which in no way are inferior to 'nouvelle cuisine'. If your body were able to talk to you it would probably advise you to follow these ten rules for healthy nutrition, which would assist you to have a long and healthy life.

Ten Rules for Healthy Eating

1. The main part of the food should be of plant origin. Fruit, vegetables and salads should, with grain products and potatoes, be the basis of nutrition. This plant nutrition should take up at least 70 per cent of the entire intake of food. In this way a high fibre content is guaranteed, which is absolutely essential for your digestion.

2. Raw, uncooked food should be not the exception, but an important part of your daily nutrition. When half of our food is of plant origin and is eaten raw, this is excellent for our health. When there is no inflammation of the intestines, more of this kind of food can be eaten.

3. Meat, poultry and fish should, as a general rule, be only eaten once a week. One can give these up for long periods without problems.

4. The proportion of fat in food should be not more than 20–30 per cent. Animal fat should be avoided as much as possible. Instead, plant fats (unsaturated oils) should be used.

5. The more natural the food is (this means not industrially prefabricated), the better it is.

6. You should live completely, or almost completely, without sugar. General rule: use no more sugar than salt.

7. There should be long intervals between meals. General rule: five hours. Longer intervals will never harm you.

8. Sour milk products are much better than regular milk products.

9. Drink plenty. Water or herb teas are ideal drinks. Lemonades or juices should be avoided.

10. Alcohol should only be drunk in small quantities.

Most of these recommendations will probably seem logical to you. These rules should become a daily routine and a matter of course, so I will deal with them in greater depth.

Rules One and Two

The right nutrition is as natural as possible. Food from plants is medicine for the body.

Vegetarian products have been, for the entire history of the human race, the main calorie donors. They are available at all times and can be prepared without much problem. Animals run away, plants don't. We have become adjusted to them. Therefore, the most important part of our nutrition should be fresh vegetables, salads, fruit, grains, potatoes, herbs, nuts and legumes. In principle, all vegetarian products can be recommended. Only a few of them are difficult to digest (for example, stone fruits and legumes). It has been proven that raw food is especially good for you when eaten at the start of a meal, and provides immense saturation value.

Wholemeal products should have an outstanding position in a healthy diet. On average they contain about ten times as much indigestible fibre as fruit and vegetables. Therefore, under normal circumstances the easiest way to meet the need for fibre is to eat wholemeal products. To put this another way, there are about 20 grams of fibre in 1 kilogram of fruit, and in 100 grams of crispbread.

Through eating nothing but vegetables, fruit and grain products, it is possible to receive all the vitamins one needs. These vegetarian foods also contain so-called secondary vegetable substances, which lower blood pressure, prevent infections, increase immune defences and even help to prevent cancer! Unfortunately, during the last years the environmental situation has changed so drastically that healthy living should also include 'toxin-free' nutrition. To live completely free of environmental toxins is not possible anymore, as even in the Antarctic pesticides are found. Major worldwide and political changes need to be made to have any effect, but this is no reason for resignation. On the contrary, healthy nutrition becomes even more important.

Although it is impossible to prevent the assimilation of certain poisons, the quantity is under your own influence. Therefore, when shopping you should pay attention to what you are purchasing. Whenever possible you should buy products of organic cultivation. At least some of the dangerous toxins (for example nitrates) will not be in these products, or only in very small quantities. Substances sprayed over wide areas do not stop outside the boundaries of a farmer who has organic cultivation. Even though he himself does not spray his crops with those, look where those products are coming from. In some countries there is a rigorous use of pesticides and fertilisers. In Germany (and this is not nationalism), this use is not too bad. Instead of imported foods it is better to buy local vegetables of the corresponding season and region. Besides, seen from an ecological point of view it is unfavourable to transport food on a truck over long distances. Every kind of food in Germany has an average transport distance of over 284 km! When buying fruit, if you keep to fruit and vegetables of the corresponding season you will reduce the assimilation of toxins, as hothouse products are usually more contaminated than products of the land. Especially problematic are salads which have a great surface, such as lettuce, spinach, iceberg lettuce and endive. In these products the nitrite content is very high. You should take off all the outer layers and wash them very well. It is recommended that you take out the hard ribs; these contain the most nitrates. Products with a lesser surface (such as tomatoes, onions, carrots and courgettes) take in less poisonous substances. Throw away the cooking water. Luckily, much of the toxins stay in the water.

Often, heavy metals accumulate in plants when they are grown near roads. I would mention especially celery, spinach and wild mushrooms. Cultivated mushrooms are better and spinach should only be purchased from controlled cultivations. By washing and peeling the pollution can be greatly reduced. When fruit has a smooth surface (such as apples) a firm rub with a cloth is just as effective as peeling.

Rule Three

Meat, poultry and fish should be eaten at the most once a week.

Meat has never been the main source of nutrition for the human being. Romantic ideas from the hunter and gatherer period, or from the 'old Teutons' gnawing on haunches of venison, are without any foundation. On the contrary, today's meat consumption beats all records. However, one kind of meat is not the same as another. Much depends on the quality. Nowadays when eating meat, we absorb many undesirable substances. These are unwelcome and can produce diseases (e.g. arteriosclerosis, gout and disturbances in the digestion of fats). Therefore one, or at the most, two meals per week which include meat is a guide that one should stick to. If you are used to a daily meat consumption, certain changes are necessary. However, after a period of time you will not miss it anymore. There is no need to eat meat. If you want to, you can do without meat altogether. You can get protein in other ways. Grains, for example, contain valuable protein. By combining grains with yogurt or curd cheese this value can be improved upon. The combination of milk protein and wheat has a higher biological value than beef with potatoes.

If you never eat meat, it would be advisable once in a while to have your blood checked for iron deficiency.

When you do not eat any meat, milk products or eggs you will have to choose your nutrition very carefully. Often deficiencies are found in this kind of diet. This is especially true for women who lose much blood during menstruation; they often need more iron. For them it is sometimes necessary to take iron tablets. But there is no reason to worry about this. Rye bread contains just as much iron as beef (ca: 3.2 mg-/100 gr).

When consuming comparatively little meat, you can circumvent most problems concerning animal protein. You should also bear the following in mind: avoid – as far as possible – meat from intensive livestock farming. Under such circumstances, shredders use medicaments (antibiotics, hormones, vitamins) on a wider scale in order to minimise the risk of disease, which this kind of breeding may provoke. Pigs and calves are especially prone to contamination. Because of this, you should avoid pork. Eat the innards of these animals as little as possible (also those of game). Here, all residues of drugs and toxins accumulate. Innards are collectors of a high level of uric acid. This is due to an uncontrolled use of vitamins during breeding. Liver often contains great quantities of vitamin A. Therefore, pregnant women should avoid eating liver. When preparing poultry from intensive farming you should make sure that the meat is thoroughly cooked. These animals are often loaded with salmonella. Only when there is adequate heat will those germs be killed. If possible let poultry defrost in the refrigerator, and do not put it on a porous base (e.g. on a wooden or plastic board). Germs are attracted to these types of surface. Smooth materials like porcelain and marble are much more hygienic.

When buying fish you should preferably choose lean sea fish, or freshwater fish, living in unpolluted water (for example trout). Fish is an excellent alternative to meat.

My advice concerning eggs, which also belong to the group of animal proteins, would be to limit oneself to 2–3 eggs per week. In this way the intake of too much cholesterol will be prevented. Those of you who do not want to go without eggs can now buy several yolk-free diet products and with these one can make scrambled eggs, omelettes and other egg dishes. They contain practically no cholesterol.

Rule Four

The proportion of fat in food should be not more than 20–30 per cent. Vegetable fats are better than animal fat.

As you were told, fat consumption in Europe and the United States is very high and what is even worse is that, by mainly eating animal fat, our organism is greatly over-burdened. Do not consume more than 80 grams of fat per day. Those fats should mainly come from plants with a high content of unsaturated fatty acids, for example wheat-germ oil. These unsaturated oils are very good when used in salads. Please remember that these highly valuable cold-pressed oils can be preserved for only one or two months and they should be stored away from the light. They are unsuitable for frying, as when heated they change into saturated oils. It is quite possible that during this transition some intermediate stages can be produced which are dangerous for health. Therefore, when frying your food it is better to use saturated oil, e.g. olive oil, or special dietary products.

Often the question is asked, which is healthier, margarine or butter? However, it is much more important to know that sausages are something which should never be eaten. They not only contain lots of animal fat, but also many residues from the animals' innards. Alternatives are soya spreads, poultry sausages or poultry ham.

In order to reduce cholesterol in the blood, the previously mentioned roughage is important. The fibre of oats, beans and special pectins are said to be very favourable. In the case of wheat, this seems to be less important.

Rule Five

The more natural the food is, the better it is. Ready-made food should be eaten as seldom as possible. However, not everything made by the industry has to be inferior. Many deep-freeze products are equivalent to fresh food. However, when buying the customary ready-made food, then certainly you will eat one of the following substances: artificial colourings; substances for anti-oxidation; preservatives; emulsifiers; thickeners; gelling agents; taste strengtheners; acid agents; acid regulators; separating agents; modified starches; artificial sweeteners; dough-raising agents; agents to prevent foam; substances for treating the flour, and more.

Moreover, these are only the different categories of additives. Behind every name there are many hidden substances; it is impossible to know them all. Some of them perhaps are harmless, but others are more harmful. About the complicated interaction of these substances, we know very little.

Almost all ready-made products are prepared with a great deal of salt. In this way the food will be preserved and it tastes right. Salt, however, is a real risk factor in the development of high blood pressure, as is nitrate (pickled foods) and sulphate (dried fruit). Sweet wine you can easily do without. Spices, on the contrary, you can eat without problem. They stimulate the digestion of your food. With glutamate, which is used as a taste strengthener, however, you do need to be careful.

Rule Six

You should live completely, or almost completely, without sugar. It would be advisable to give up sugar completely.

Alas! Avoiding sugar is very difficult for most people. Still, this is a very important, maybe the most important, step towards healthy eating. Sugar is a concentrated food which only gives you 'empty calories'. Our organism has in no way been prepared for such an artificial food.

When you eat sugar, the organism misses the original substances which were taken out in the course of the production processes. This is not only the roughage, but also the vitamins and trace elements. Vitamins are especially essential as they are needed to assist in the assimilation and the utilisation of the sugar in the body. Therefore, when you eat sugar vitamin deposits in the body will be used and you will be lacking in vitamins (especially vitamin B complex). Because of this, sugar is often called 'a vitamin thief'.

When eating a bar of chocolate you actually ingest the energy value (calories) of one sugar beet. The body, during human development, was not used to such a compact quantity of energy and so it still thinks that it is getting the entire sugar beet and not the condensed version. Therefore, it starts producing great quantities of acids and enzymes in order to assimilate the non-existent sugar beet (mainly the fibres therein). In the end these digestive juices irritate the digestive channels, as they cannot find the corresponding food and are superfluous. Moreover, such concentrated food gives only a very short-lived feeling of saturation. Eating one sugar beet could probably satisfy you more, but a chocolate bar only satisfies you for a short while. The feeling of saturation depends on the number of calories as well as on the volume of the food. So when calories are separated from volume, you really have to eat more in order to feel saturated. This is the real cause of the widespread obesity problem. It is, on the contrary, extremely difficult to gain weight whilst eating only natural products.

Sugar is, for the organism, not just 'one of these things'. Sugar, or to be more exact, glucose, is the final product of the entire digestion of carbohydrate. Potatoes, bread and fruit are changed into glucose by different intermediate stages. When sugar is supplied direct there is no need for the entire process of digestion, because in a chemical 'short circuit' sugar goes straight into the bloodstream. This is probably the cause of the urge to eat sugar. It is one substance that one does not need to get used to slowly. Therefore, it is logical that one can get addicted to sugar.

Such behaviour hardly differs from nicotine or alcohol addiction. This you can easily prove for yourself. Do you absolutely need to have some sugar (to eat something sweet)? Does this happen every day? Do you always keep something sweet in the house? Does it ever happen that you turn the house upside down in order to find a piece of chocolate? Do you sometimes go out just to buy something sweet? Do you get up during the night to nibble something sweet? If you are aware of this kind of behaviour in yourself, then sugar addiction is quite possible. Especially in the case of children, sugar addiction is wide-spread on a frightening scale. Such children very often need something sweet, otherwise they become bad tempered, sad or depressed. Immediately after eating a piece of chocolate their mood changes and they are completely happy again. Such a phenomenon is well known in other kinds of addiction.

Accordingly, during the weaning off sugar there are withdrawal symptoms; sudden attacks of a craving for sugar can be accompanied by a feeling of weakness or by perspiring; patients regularly tell me they feel irritated or depressed. Luckily, this period of transition only takes a short time. After a week, the strongest symptoms are done with. The appetite for sugar, the subjective seduction, however, takes longer. But after a couple of months at the most the person in question will look more relaxed when other people eat chocolate or pastries. However, when you again start to eat sweets the addiction returns.

If you have decided not to eat any more sugar, people will not make it easy for you. First you will have to learn how to recognise sugar-free foods. When it says 'sugar-free' or 'without sugar', this will not always mean that there is really no sugar in the food. Often it just means that the product does not contain any sugar emanating from sugar beets. Also, the producers are learning, and therefore they use other kinds of sugar, which provides better publicity.

There are innumerable kinds of sugar. Seen from a biological viewpoint, all of them provoke more or less the same reaction. They are all 'empty calories' for which the organism was never made. Also, the information 'suitable for diabetics' does not mean that it is harmless. It just means that in order to digest it no insulin is needed. This, however, has little to do with the real harm that sugar can do to your health. Other kinds of sugar contain just as many calories and harm the digestion and the teeth just as much, in the same way. Some sweeteners (orbit, xylem, isomalt) also give wind or act as a laxative.

Sugar can be in the following forms:

household sugar	maple syrup
crystal sugar	corn syrup
refined sugar	malt dextrine
powdered sugar	malt sugar
brown sugar	milk sugar
cane sugar	maltose
succonate	lactose
molasses	fructose
beet sugar	asorbic
sugar beet sugar	mannit
	isomalt

Honey is not an artificial product. However, it does contain 80 per cent sugar (invert sugar)! Sadly, many people who want to eat healthily tend to overlook this. Therefore, honey is no substitute for sugar. In small quantities (as a condiment) it can be used without any harmful effects. The same is true for brown sugar, which consists of 90 per cent saccaroses (household sugar). Molasses also contains 60 per cent sugar, as well as some unwanted substances from the sugar beets. Those few good substances which can be found in honey, brown sugar and molasses (traces of vitamins) you can just as well get from other kinds of food. In order to get enough of these quantities one would, in this case, have to eat great portions of these sweet calorific substances.

Sweeteners do not have calories. Their digestion is different. We do not know anything about their harmful effects. However, in the case of two of those (saccharine and cyclamate) the risk of cancer (when taken in high quantities) might be a possibility. For aspartin, nothing is known about cancer risk. In the body aspartin is broken down by way of the intermediate stage of methanol and formaldehyde. These two substances have recently been regarded as responsible for addictive behaviour.

In small quantities, sweeteners aid the change to sugar-free nutrition, or to nutrition with very little sugar, by making it easier. However, sweeteners are not unproblematic and you should not use unlimited quantities. If you want to save on calories they are not very helpful, because sweeteners increase appetite. Although they do not contain any fuel for the body, using them makes the food taste better and therefore you will eat more. People who regularly use sweeteners, therefore, in the final analysis do not take in less calories. There is no other way – you have to discover the original taste of the food, without covering this up with sugar or sweeteners. After a short time, you will be amazed to discover how much more interesting food can be.

Rule Seven

There should be long intervals between meals.

In the number of meals, less is better. Maybe you will be surprised when I tell you that it is better to observe intervals between meals. Probably you have often heard that it is better to eat as many small meals as possible. When given this advice, it is often overlooked that food stays for a certain length of time in the stomach. A mixed meal leaves the stomach after 4–5 hours. If, before this time, new food comes into the stomach, it is mixed with the food which is already there and there are now two possibilities: the food stays in the stomach as long as it takes for the second addition to be well digested. In that case, the first meal starts fermenting in the stomach. As a second possibility, no consideration is taken of the newly arrived food and everything is immediately pushed into the intestines. In that case, the second portion is not prepared at all, or is only prepared partly, for further digestion. Therefore, bacteria in the small intestine will decompose the food and as a result there are fermentation symptoms, this time in the small intestine.

Often, decisions to eat small meals divided over the day have not been thought over seriously. Many people feel, at the latest two or three hours after a meal, the urge to eat something, as otherwise they will be troubled by a sudden craving for food, feelings of weakness, a decrease of blood pressure or perspiring. This is a vicious circle and fermentation in the stomach is the actual cause of these problems.

Changing these kinds of eating habits is usually somewhat easier than abstaining from sugar. It is advisable, especially if in the beginning there is a feeling of weakness, to drink plenty. Bitter-tasting teas, such as vermouth or fennel tea, have been known to be helpful. When this rhythm is changed, after a few weeks no more feelings of weakness will occur. Instead, many people learn for the first time in their lives what it means to feel really hungry. Up until then, this feeling will have been confused with indisposition or weakness and, finally, there will be no noise from the stomach. Real hunger does not have anything to do with such symptoms.

By eating three meals, in so far as those meals follow the prescribed course, the blood-sugar levels can be well balanced. Now the stomach will deliver the food at regular intervals into the intestines and the fibres will take care that the food is slowly assimilated. There is no problem if you prefer to eat even less often; when eating only one or two meals a day, one can live well. However, there is always this condition. Only by eating food (vegetables, raw vegetables, wholemeal products) which is difficult to break down can a sudden massive flooding of food into the digestive system and into the blood be prevented. This knowledge about the right frequency of meals is nothing new. Many people feel that this is the right way and automatically they do not eat anything between meals. In many great civilisations this was the usual custom. However, in case you should have any doubts, you can experiment over the course of a few days and eat as diabetics are often forced to do. During the course of a few days you will eat seven meals a day and observe how you feel. The principle of having intervals between meals should be recommended for most diabetic patients, and later on I will tell you more about this.

Rule Eight

Sour milk products are better than regular milk products.

Milk's good reputation is deceptive. Milk is, strictly speaking, the only adequate food. Newborn children make do with it exclusively over a long period of time. From all sides, the advantages of milk are praised. Calcium, phosphorus, vitamins, protein – you can find everything in milk. There is nothing wrong with this. However, whole milk has some disadvantages.

Again I have to go back to the history of our development. During the longest period of our history we did not ingest any milk, with the exception of mother's milk. Therefore, after the age of adulthood there was no need to continue the production of enzymes (mainly lactose, needed for the digestion of milk) and the production of these enzymes in the course of childhood was discontinued. These days this situation has hardly changed. Most people in the world do not have any lactose available after childhood. Therefore, people from Asia and Africa do not drink milk. They do not tolerate milk and promptly get stomach-aches when they take it. The Chinese think that a glass of milk is a terrible thing, as to them it is a glass of cow saliva.

When people who do not have enough of these enzymes drink whole cow's milk, they get diarrhoea right away. This, however, does not apply to acid milk products. Here, bacteria has already broken down the problematic milk sugar. In Europe, especially in northern and middle Europe, we have a special situation. Those who live in the north have more lactose in their bodies. People in Scandinavia have up to 90 per cent sufficient enzymes to break down milk sugar and therefore tolerate milk quite well. In the German-speaking countries, this percentage is much lower. Forty per cent of the people there do not tolerate milk. This situation is much worse in the Mediterranean countries, where many of the population do not have the necessary enzymes for milk digestion.

This north-south divide has an interesting background. The causes of it are the different grades of sun rays, and calcium metabolism. An important requirement for the healthy development of the bones in a child is sufficient calcium supply. As there is an abundance of calcium in plants, when a child eats sufficient vegetables and salads there will be no deficiency symptoms. However, the assimilation of calcium in the body is tied to two other conditions: there should be enough vitamin D available, and there should be plenty of sunlight on the skin, as this changes vitamin D into its usable form. These conditions are fulfilled in southern countries. No lack of calcium is known there. In the north the situation is different. Only in summer is there enough sunshine. Vegetables and fruit are scarce. There is a danger of lack of calcium and of developing rickets. In this situation, an added calcium supply through milk is a blessing. Those people who could digest milk products (also fresh milk) were fortunate. During the colonisation of northern Europe, the hereditary factor of lactose, therefore, was a great selective advantage. Within a few thousand years the corresponding gene spread through people living there and it is still the same in the present day.

You will be able to tell if you yourself have enough lactose at your disposal. When there is a marked lack of this enzyme, after drinking a glass of milk, or, for example, when you eat ice-cream, you will get excessive wind or you will have diarrhoea. When there is only a slight lack of lactose, symptoms are less noticeable. Furthermore, you must realise that many foods contain milk. Therefore, stomach-aches can occur on many different occasions and this makes a clear diagnosis very difficult. Some people only find out what has been bothering them for their entire lifetime when they are quite old. Therefore, when you are not sure it seems best to refrain from drinking whole milk.

Fermented or sour milk products (for example acidic milk or curd cheese) can be tolerated, as the milk sugar which gives most problems has been dealt with by bacteria. Therefore, Africans, Chinese and Indians can tolerate sour milk products quite well. Generally the left-turning (in its processing) kind (L+) is best and should be favoured. Right-turning acid milk could, if used in greater quantities (more than 1 kg per day), lead to a hyper-acidity of the blood.

I repeat, you should not only avoid regular milk – I also mean low-fat cow's milk. Cream, butter or cheese are usually better tolerated, as milk sugar is soluble in water and these products contain very little milk sugar. Acid milk products can be recommended, as they are favourable for the intestinal bacteria.

Besides people with a lack of lactose, those with a tendency to allergies should be careful concerning milk. You will probably know that some foods can provoke allergies. Milk is top of the list; 42 per cent of all food allergies are triggered by milk, and it may take years or decades before this is discovered in a patient. The reason that milk can be so allergy-provoking is baby-feeding habits. After mother's milk, cow's milk is usually the first strange food that a baby comes into contact with. However, the intestines of a baby are different to the intestines of an adult. A baby can absorb the big protein-building blocks of milk without breaking them down first. The baby can use valuable substances for this defence from the mother's milk. However, this mechanism turns out to be very unfavourable when the baby is fed cow's milk. The protein-building blocks from the cow's milk are still absorbed, but they are recognised as foreign matter. The baby starts to produce anti-bodies against cow's milk. In special cases the baby gets a 'scaly-skin' disease, which comes from the incompatibility of cow's milk.

Therefore, feeding the baby yourself is the best protection against allergies. It seems that mother's milk not only helps against food allergies but also prevents or reduces other kinds of allergies. This is especially important when there are already allergic tendencies in the family. In that case, adding eggs and fish to the baby's diet should be postponed as long as possible. Those foods often trigger incompatibilities.

Something important – people with stomach problems often like to drink milk, as milk binds the surplus acid. However, for a while it has been known that after binding the acids, a very high production of hydrochloric acid will start, which in its intensity is only surpassed by alcohol. The patient who is tormented by stomach-aches, again starts to drink milk, which will for only a short period of time give him some relief.

Someone who does not like to do without milk should try as an alternative the unsweetened soya milk. This is made from ground soy beans and water under application of steam and it becomes a milk-like drink, which is well known in Asiatic countries.

However, a person who is not allergic and has no stomach problems and finally does not lack lactose, can drink milk without any problem. In this case one should realise that milk is not a drink, but a meal. So do not drink milk as a thirst-quencher between meals.

Rule Nine

Drink plenty – the best is water. It is good to drink plenty. You need about two litres of liquid daily as an average quantity. When the weather is warm, or when you do physical exercise, this quantity can be increased to three litres or even more. Tiredness or fatigue, especially when sitting at a desk, is often caused by a lack of liquid. In that case coffee only helps temporarily, and at the same time kidney function is stimulated and therefore more liquid will be eliminated.

The ideal drink for human beings is water. As clean, uncontaminated water from the tap, mineral water or herbal tea, this is the best way to recompense loss of liquid. In the infrastructure of food refinement, the importance of water has been diminished. Lemonades and juices have been established as thirst quenching. The increase in the consumption of these is impressive. Between 1950 and 1988 there was an increase of 750 per cent. Children, especially, are often used to drinking juices or soft drinks to supply the daily need for liquids. Generally, those are considered healthy as they contain vitamins and come from natural products. However, apple juice cannot be compared to an apple, and sugar in no way to sugar beets! The roughage and fibre are lacking, the things which make an apple a healthy product. The digestive tract is fooled by these substances, which lack exactly those ingredients which help to develop peristaltic movements.

Ease of consumption is paid for with a growing tiredness of the intestinal muscles. Think about how many apples or oranges you would have to squeeze in order to obtain one full bottle of juice. You could probably drink such a bottle easily in the course of an evening – as an extra. However, you would never be able to eat all of the original fruit – very soon you would be over saturated. The number of calories stays about the same. You have been fooling your feelings of saturation with this juice, and it is the same with all concentrated food or drink. You can eat lots of fruit, but eat it in its natural state. The more work of chewing, swallowing and digestion there is, the healthier you will become. The teeth become stronger, the gums are massaged and the intestines receive much-needed fibre material.

This rule applies even more to lemonades. Their sugar content is higher. Valuable substances are hardly found at all. Vitamins are added at the most as a selling point. Those drinks you can forget about. With the right kind of food, as I explained to you, your body will get more than enough vitamins.

Rule Ten

Alcohol should only be drunk in small quantities.

Alcohol has quite a long tradition in our culture. In the past people liked to drink during festivities and sometimes they drank excessively. However, following the festivities there were long periods when there were no financial means to afford this 'party-drinking'. All this has changed, with other foods 'for special occasions'. In the meantime, beer, wine and other alcoholic drinks have become part of daily pleasure. They are served all the time and everywhere. Statistics of the last 40 years show us this growing tendency. The consumption of strong alcoholic beverages has increased threefold. The quantity of beer drunk has increased by four times and people now drink five times as much wine as before. The consequences are known.

Alcohol in small quantities is not harmful to healthy adults. There are many controversial ideas about how much one should drink. At the most, 20–40 gmme of alcohol per day (for example two glasses of wine) should be drunk. This limit should not be exceeded. It is best not to drink alcohol every day. Your liver needs a rest in order to recover. These limits are meant for men – a woman's liver does not tolerate alcohol as well as a man's. It should be mentioned that the 'unharmful' quantity of alcohol, has been lowered each year. It is quite possible that in the future alcohol will be seen in a more critical light.

First steps to follow in case of digestive problems

Maybe, after reading this book, you will decide to change your nutritional habits. You'll decide to follow the ten rules for healthy eating and after a short time you feel happy and have excellent results. After eating you feel really satisfied, without any burping or feeling of being filled to the brim.

Until the next meal, you are not conscious of your stomach. On the contrary, there prevails a state of complete well-being which is difficult to describe. When your stomach calls your attention there is a feeling of real hunger, which has nothing to do with weakness. Your bowel movement is punctual, the stool is voluminous and soft. Above all, you feel full of energy and full of life. If you previously had a comparatively healthy digestive system, you will make this change without any important physical problems. If this applies to you, you can skip the chapter on digestion.

Unfortunately, in most cases this is not the case. When for a period of years – maybe all your life – you have eaten the 'normal' nutrition of civilisation, the demands made on your stomach have been very little, causing the muscles of the digestive tract to become weak, as they have never, in a biological way, been sufficiently challenged. When an intestine which has for many years been coddled in this way, is confronted all of a sudden with labour-demanding natural food, it seems logical that there will be problems of transition. This resembles the situation when an inactive man, on the spur of the moment, decides to become sporty and right away starts running ten miles. Immediately following the first try, he will feel so bad that he prefers to continue living an easy life. People who start eating healthily without having any training often relate the following: 'I tried to eat healthy coarse whole bread, fresh salads, muesli and all this did not agree with me. I got stomach-aches and, above all, terrible flatulence.' These and similar reports all clearly show that the digestive system of the people concerned is untrained and that there are probably inflammations. So, in that case, coarse food passes too fast through the small intestine.

As long as the only food eaten is easy to digest these symptoms are seldom noticed, as in that case the food concentrates enter into the blood at a faster rate. But the coarser food comes into the blood at a slower rate. Now, it passes by the inflamed surface of the upper part of the intestines and comes into the deeper-lying sections. These sections are less suited to metabolic changes and here a special kind of bacteria can, because of the much bigger food supply, multiply extensively. This kind of bacteria is responsible for the development of gases (fermentation).

What to do now? Many people come to the conclusion 'natural food does not agree with me', and they again start to eat the food that they are used to. Of course, the inflammation will not disappear but will just be felt less. In the long run, this problem worsens. The alternative solution is a slow transition from the food one is used to eating to a healthier way of eating – a reconstruction of nutrition.

When changing your diet, you have to keep in mind that you must adjust slowly, as your digestive tract will still be relatively irritated. Then, when the inflammation lessens, higher demands can be made of the peristaltic muscles until gradually a new equilibrium is reached. In the same way, during a training programme for the muscles of the skeleton one starts with little stress. Then the demands on the muscles of the intestines can increase (jogging of the intestine). The better the situation is at the beginning (few symptoms, mild discomfort), the shorter the first phase will be. However, when there are serious problems, the need for careful treatment is extremely important, as the entire digestive system should be regenerated.

A LIGHT AND SPECIAL DIET

In the stage of training, you should be able to reach two different goals: the irritation of the intestines should be healed through eating a light and special diet, and at the same time the intestines should be prepared for the digestion of bigger quantities of the right food, rich in fibre.

For a long time, eating light food meant eating oat gruel, rice gruel, semolina or tea and toast. The common factor of this kind of food rests with the boiling and also the long baking of cereals.

Why has such nutrition been used for thousands of years in the treatment of stomach irritation? During the process of cooking cereals, the structure of their molecules is changed. Carbohydrates have naturally long molecules. During the cooking process they form a kind of network whereby a mucus-like slime is produced. In the digestive tract, this slime coats the entire inner skin, like a thin film. Under this protective skin it is possible for the surface of the intestines to heal and to renew itself.

With the help of this 'inner protective skin' the inflamed parts can be cured. Medication (e.g. H2 blocker) should not be used at this time. It is true that this kind of medication is able to decrease the symptoms within a short time, but as soon as it is not taken anymore the old problems reappear. The medication only suppresses the production of acids. However, acids are not the real cause of the inflammation of the stomach; the acidity is only an after-effect. It would seem more logical to stop the symptoms, while at the same time protect the stomach walls so that healing is possible.

How should this special diet be prepared? First, you

grind cereals. Depending on your taste and what is available, you will have a choice of wheat, rye, oats, barley, buckwheat, millet, quinoa and other cereals or mixtures of those. This coarsely ground cereal should be boiled until it resembles a soup or a porridge and there are no more hard parts to be found. This usually takes 15 to 30 minutes, depending on how finely the cereal has been shredded. One thing is most important: the more serious the inflammation and subsequently the symptoms, the softer and more slimy the food should be. The cereals can be soaked in water overnight (e.g. in the refrigerator), where they will swell up and be more easily digested. As a foundation for the soup I recommend the use of a vegetable broth, which can be made at home or bought ready made in a health food store. There are good products available, for example with a base of yeast. It is important that only clear broth is used as a base, as any additions could irritate the stomach.

This soup or porridge, prepared three times a day, should be the only nutrition during the first stage of the diet. Depending on the kind of problem, this first stage can last a few days, up to three weeks or even longer. This will not be easy. In the beginning, certainly, it is a little difficult. However, you will very quickly get used to this new food, especially when you see the first results.

In case these recommendations seem very far-fetched to you, please think about the diets of the Romans and the Teutons. For thousands of years porridge and soup were their daily basic nutrition. These were the forerunners of our bread and were eaten for a much longer time. In other parts of the world, it is certain that nobody would be surprised about your nutrition. So, seen from a historical and geographical point of view, you will find yourself in good company! By doing this for a while you will go back to our original way of nutrition.

In order that the food tastes good to you, it will be worthwhile to use some imagination while preparing it. A spring soup, Italian soup, different kinds of broth, also sometimes just a clear meat broth, can provide some variation. The quantity depends on your appetite. Please eat until you are satisfied. Generally those quantities lie between 50 and 120g cereal per meal. Young men or teenagers sometimes need more. Even when you are satisfied with this quantity, you will not gain but will lose weight. Often this is a much desired side-effect. Some overweight people can lose up to ten kg in three weeks. In case you do not want to lose weight, but still want to cure the problems of the intestinal tract, you may add some fat (butter, cream, oil) to the soup or the porridge. As you know, fat is assimilated by way of the lymphatic system. However, this does not mean any kind of fat. Some kinds of fat get directly into the bloodstream without making the detour through the lymphatic system. These kinds of fats (oil or special margarine from the health-food shop) should be used when you do not want to lose weight, but want to relieve the lymphatic system.

Please drink plenty during this time, especially if you want to lose weight, when many different substances should be flushed out of the system. It is good to drink two litres a day, or more. It is excellent to drink special herb tea in between meals, for example when you feel hunger pangs. Fennel, chamomile, caraway, vermouth, or different mixtures of these herbs, are good. Although a bitter tea does not taste very nice, it is excellent for the digestion. I recommend you drink at least one cup of tea between meals.

The vitamin content (especially vitamin B complex) of this part of the diet is not sufficient for your needs over a long period. Also, in the cooking process many vitamins are lost. However, there will be no loss of vitamins in a short period of a few weeks. If you are taking this soup diet for a long period of time, it is good to take additional vitamins.

As an alternative to cereal soup or vegetable porridge, you can perhaps prepare a potato soup. Although potatoes contain much less roughage or protein than the cereals, they are very easily digested and are not secret fatteners – if they are not served as chips. This kind of food is absolutely right for every day.

With the different tasks and distractions of everyday life it will be easy to follow this diet, but on a holiday you may think about all the 'good things' you could be eating instead, and so it may be harder to stick to it.

You can prepare your lunch in the morning and take it with you to your work. If during this time you are losing weight, it is logical that you will suffer some symptoms. The body will try to save energy and because of this you will feel shivery, your hands and feet will be colder than normal and your blood pressure may go down a bit. As soon as your energy level is back to normal again, these symptoms will disappear completely.

The duration of this first healing and cleansing process depends on how serious your problems are. When there are only slight symptoms, it will be all right to follow this diet for one week. More serious symptoms mean that a longer diet period of one to three weeks may be necessary.

It is the same in the case of being overweight. When you eat in this way, it is easy to lose weight.

The advice I would give to overweight patients is always to eat until they feel satisfied. Because of the great saturation value of cooked cereals (swelling of grains), it is not possible to eat the same quantity of calories as before. So the weight loss follows on automatically, without the patient feeling hungry.

Of course, it is a big change to eat such a simple and strange diet, especially during the first days when it is difficult not to eat the food one has been used to. After all, eating can be a consolation, a reward or a compensation for disappointments or depression. If food for you also means inner stabilisation, as it does for many people, then you will become a little unbalanced in the beginning or maybe feel restless and irritable. My advice for these days is be good to yourself! Reward yourself for your achievement – but not by eating and drinking. Do something! It would be especially good to go somewhere that you do not have to eat – the cinema, theatre, concerts, etc. All are activities which would distract you during the evening.

It is very pleasant to diet together with other people. If you have company, it will be easier for you to stay steadfast. Partners or relatives can motivate and help one another. The goal of this light diet is the healing of the inflammation of the stomach. You will realise how the feeling of being full up slowly decreases and there will be less burping, intestinal noises and flatulence. When you are feeling better, you can start with the next phase of healthy nutrition. The most difficult time now lies behind you.

THE REBUILDING OF YOUR NUTRITIONAL PROGRAMME

Now you will probably have a great desire to eat fresh salads, fruit and vegetables. This is only natural. However, when you change straight away to eating coarse salads or fruit, many of you will have problems. These can be felt as flatulence, or a feeling of restlessness or pain in the tummy. Therefore, you need a time of adaptation in which the nutritional programme can be reconstructed. You will remember, the more the intestinal tract is irritated, the slower the change should be. There is another advantage when you are careful in this respect: when every day a new kind of food is added, it will be easy to discover eventual food allergies or incompatibilities. In this way you can learn things, which otherwise would stay hidden from observation.

For most people the following procedure is next. Start to expand your diet by eating vegetables. You should take those species which do not provoke flatulence, such as carrots, zucchini, fennel or asparagus, which are the best. These vegetables can be eaten with soup or porridge or they can be prepared as an ingredient of these. Also, potatoes (with the skin on or boiled with salt), wholegrain rice, maize with vegetables (e.g. polenta) or cereal steaks can be eaten once in a while and will replace the cereals. Generally they are tolerated quite well. Also, you can now use some butter, sour cream or oil. These things will improve the taste considerably. In a fatless meal you cannot taste substances which are only soluble in fats, and you can use some (e.g. parmesan cheese).

When you can tolerate this, you can also eat salads to

complement your nutrition. I would advise you to start with green salads (e.g. lettuce): because of their large surface in comparison to their volume, they can easily be broken down. Throw away the outer leaves and if possible use only salads which have not been treated with artificial fertilisers. Only after a while can you use the coarser salads which, however, should be cut finely and chewed well. The sauce for the salad depends on your habits and on what agrees with you – for example vinegar, oil or yogurt.

As the next step, you can start to eat bread. The easiest to digest is crispbread. Soy spreads are good and these are available in many different tastes. Soy sausages are also an excellent substitute for real meat sausages, which you should avoid. When your body is used to the crispbread, you can start eating wholemeal bread with butter and low fat cheeses. In case the coarse bread does not agree with you, you should try a very finely ground wholemeal bread. Do not be afraid to ask your baker if this bread really has been made from whole grains, even if he offers it under the title 'whole grain'. Sometimes bread with good-sounding names have nothing to do with real wholemeal bread. Often this is made from mixtures in which whole grains are only a small part, amongst many others. The dark colour has often been made by added colourings (sugar colouring or coffee). You can only be sure when the baker grinds the grains that you are buying wholemeal bread.

For breakfast you can prepare a whole grain muesli. The best muesli is made from grain you grind yourself. If this is not possible, you should go somewhere they grind it for you and use it as soon as possible. The wholemeal grains should be soaked in a little water overnight (for at least three hours). In the morning, you remove what is left from the water, add a shredded apple and after, to suit your taste, other fresh fruit. Yoghurt, thickened milk or sour milk will give the finishing touch. According to taste, you can also add some raisins, nuts, sunflower seeds or other such goods as an interesting addition. If you do not find this preparation sweet enough, you can use a small amount of sweetener. For the muesli you can use any kind of cereal – experiment to find which cereals you prefer.

Oats, especially if they are not too coarse, hardly have to be soaked, and they can taste a little bitter if they have been soaked too long. Some people worry that when soaking grains unwanted bacteria could multiply therein. Investigations have shown that at room temperature (20 °C) grains may be soaked safely for up to ten hours. If the room temperature is higher, it is better to put them in the refrigerator.

Some people cannot tolerate raw muesli. For them it is better to boil the grains in the morning. The grains have to be boiled for about 10 to 15 minutes (in a non-stick pan). When the water has evaporated the preparation will have a similar consistency to oatmeal. Then you can add fruit and yogurt. Prepared in the right way this muesli tastes wonderful and it makes an excellent base for the rest of the day. This first meal already contains a great part of the daily requirement of fibre. Therefore this fresh muesli should be eaten once a day for breakfast or for dinner.

Ready-made muesli mixtures (out of the package) are generally made with a basis of oats, and often contain sugar or great quantities of dried fruits. They are no substitute for crushed, home-made oats. These ready-made products you should fall back on occasionally, perhaps at holiday times. If you are used to drinking coffee and tolerate it well, you do not have to cut this out. For a long time coffee was considered as an enemy of the stomach. It is true that coffee stimulates the stomach to make more acids, but the extent of this has been overrated. The acid secretion only increases mildly. The same is true for most spices. Used in reasonable quantities, even cayenne pepper and red peppers hardly harm the stomach. This is good to know as you are eating a large amount of cereal and, when eaten raw, cereals protect the stomach.

If you find that you have tolerated everything quite well, you can now expand your range of nutrition. You will know what you tolerate well and what does not agree with you, as you progress step by step towards a normal diet. All the time, you can be adding more varieties of salad or vegetables to your daily menu and you will now realise how much variation there can be. Different ways of preparation and the addition of spices can create a wealth of nutritional choice.

SALADS

artichokes	asparagus	avocados
bamboo shoots	beetroot	carrots
cauliflower	celery	chicory
corn on the cob	cucumber	cut-lettuce
dandelion	endives	escarole
fennel	French beans	kohlrabi
lamb's lettuce	lettuce	marigold
mushrooms	oak leaf salad	olives
onions	palm hearts	radishes
red cabbage	red peppers	salad gherkins

sauerkraut	shallots	soya bean sprouts
sprouts	sweet green peppers	tomatoes
watercress	white cabbage	

VEGETABLES

eggplant	sorrel	sweet potatoes
leeks	celery root	horse radish
broccoli	spinach	chilli-pots
okra pots	cabbage	Chinese leaves
peas	parsley shoots	water chestnuts
vine leaves	curly kale	Brussels sprouts
savoy	courgettes	

When preparing vegetables use as little water as possible, and steam the vegetables instead of boiling. In this way you will get more vitamins.

Just as with vegetables, there are many different kinds of fruit. You will discover a great variety. Also, there are other cereal products, like wholemeal noodles or wholemeal millet, which will make a change to your menu. Have you ever tried eating fresh bean sprouts? In two to three days you can grow sufficient (1–2mm), and these are a delicacy in salads. Besides, their vitamin content increases whilst sprouting!

In general, you should learn to be flexible with your nutrition and to react to your own feelings. When you have problems you can fall back on the first special diet and afterwards start building up your menu again. Sometimes discomfort can go quickly. When the complaints are not serious, it will be sufficient to eat cereals only for one entire day and after this to extend your menu again. However, if you suffer from a serious intestinal illness, you should eat the cereals for longer. The further you progress with your personal diet, the more difficult it will become to take advice from others. You have to monitor the reactions of your own body and get to know them. Hopefully you will be helped by following the principles shown in this book and using the ten rules as a guideline.

To end this section, I want to summarise the special diet and the rebuilding of health.

A light and special diet Cereal porridge or cereal soup and, once in a while, rice and potatoes.

The rebuilding of the nutrition You can add vegetables such as zucchini, carrots and fennel to the soup or the porridge.

Leafy salads (lettuce, lamb's lettuce) and crispbread with soya spreads.

Wholemeal bread (ground finely) with lean, hard cheese, apples and other fruit. Muesli (in the beginning with cooked cereals and natural yoghurt).

Coarser food, (coarse wholemeal) bread, fresh cereal, muesli, a great percentage of raw food, other kinds of cheese.

Expand your menu while paying attention to the ten rules.

About 6,000 years ago the Egyptians planted the first cereals, beans and many kinds of vegetables. With goats, sheep and donkeys, simple stockbreeding began. Meat was available only when an animal had to be slaughtered and was always regarded as a luxury. As an alternative, people occasionally ate fish or small game.

The main meal always consisted of gruel or porridge prepared with coarsely ground cereals, eaten with beans, onions and other vegetables. By mixing the flour with water and allowing this to dry on stones in the sun, the cereal was sometimes used to make simple 'flat-cakes'. People drank water or water mixed with a little vinegar, which was made from fermented fruit. This was an excellent thirst-quencher and was also used as a remedy for some health problems. The Egyptians already knew how to brew a simple kind of beer. Dates and other fruits were appreciated as sweets.

In the course of time, as agriculture and stockbreeding developed more fully, there was a wider choice of food, but cereals remained the principal food throughout the Middle Ages and almost up to the present time. Most people were poor and could afford only the bare necessities of life. They worked many hours a day and were obliged to give the greater part of their harvest to the big landowners. With the exception of Sundays and special holidays, they ate no meat. Most of their food was still hard and full of fibre, but because of eating this simple food, working hard and being outside in the fresh air most of the day, these people were rarely ill.

In Roman times, the lifestyle of the rich upper classes was totally different. At the many festive occasions, to which hundreds of guests were invited, they ate abundant meals, which consisted of many courses and exotic dishes. Vast quantities of meat, venison and poultry were consumed and there was no shortage of wine and other drinks. At that time wine was diluted with water, as undiluted wine was considered to be a drink for 'barbarians'.

Such rich meals were considered a status symbol and were a sign of class-consciousness. Therefore, many members of the upper classes suffered from gluttony and often became chronically ill. Thus in former times a small section of the population suffered from diseases similar to the diseases from which the majority of patients suffer today.

CEREALS AS THE MOST IMPORTANT FOOD

When nomadic tribes and cave dwellers were becoming farmers, cereals became more and more important and gradually conquered the different continents. Cereals are an excellent food for mankind as they contain carbohydrates (61 per cent), protein (15 per cent) and fat (2 per cent), as well as vitamins, minerals and many other vital elements in the right proportions.

Wholemeal cereals are a natural and nourishing food which is inexpensive and very resistant to decay. Each kind of cereal has its own characteristics and contains different nutrients, which are dependent on the climate and the properties of the soil. Rice is the main food of the East. Corn (maize) is the most important food of the West. Oats are eaten mostly in the polar latitudes and millet is the main cereal of Africa and the grasslands. The people of central Europe have always had a preference for wheat, rye and barley. Wholemeal cereals are extremely healthy; they disperse their regenerative nutrients to every part of the body.

It is even better to combine cereals with vegetables, as these improve the nutritional value still more. The combination of different raw and cooked vegetables, as was customary in old times, is excellent. Raw, whole cereal grains are a 'living food' as, even after thousands of years, if stored correctly they can still germinate.

For about 6,000 years people ate mainly oats, corn, millet, buckwheat and other cereals. After the harvest the grains were dried a little and then beaten in such a way that the husk was gradually separated from the corn and could be passed through a sieve. During this procedure the cornstarch changed into a kind of sugar, which contained all the valuable healthy ingredients. The grain was made into gruel or porridge by mixing the coarse flour with water which, without being cooked, had a sweet and succulent taste.

Rice in Asia, millet in Africa and barley, oats, wheat and millet in Europe have been treated in this way, so that the 'life-giving' substances of the grain could be preserved. To change the menu somewhat, the so-called 'flat-cakes', which people still eat in Egypt and some other countries, were made from thin layers of unfermented dough and baked in the sun. Later, such cakes were baked in the oven, very much like Mexican enchiladas and tacos or Scandinavian 'Knäckebrot'. From the Italian cuisine we know a humid, good-tasting gruel called 'polenta'. In former times everybody used freshly ground cereals, or people chewed the roasted grains, sometimes adding a little salt to make them tasty.

In the beginning, when cereals were ground, the result

was a mixture of fine and rough substances. This was good for the teeth and the digestive system. The Greeks as well as the Romans all ate barley and wheat, but as civilisation developed and more people moved into the towns, nutritional habits changed. Barley became the food of the poor people and the army, but the rich upper classes preferred to eat wheat. Wheat is a cereal which is easily digested and is much appreciated because of the many ways in which it can be used. It permits the production of the finest flour, which serves to make refined and exquisite pastries.

As in the decadent times of the Greeks and Romans before their decline, today most people prefer to eat wheat and fail to realise that any kind of refined flour is a vitamin and mineral 'robber', as is our refined white sugar. So it is no surprise that in those ancient times the rich upper classes suffered from diseases similar to those we are familiar with today.

FORMER CIVILISATIONS, THEIR RISE, GOLDEN AGE AND DECLINE

The nutrition and lifestyles of the ancient Egyptians, Greeks and Romans were similar. At first, there was hardly any difference between the rich and the poor and nearly every family owned some land, where they grew cereals and other food. When towns gradually developed, the citizens of these towns, even the mayor and the scholars, still remained farmers and continued to cultivate their own fields. Their way of eating and lifestyle remained simple until much later. They ate raw and cooked vegetables, especially onions, together with their gruel or cereal soup. Later they added other simple foods such as cheese from goats or sheep, olives, honey, figs, almonds and sometimes fish or poultry to their diet.

Gradually these ancient civilisations became more powerful The development of civilisations is always a phenomenon which in itself is limited. If we take the trouble to study world history thoroughly, we find that this was the fate of every civilisation of the Western world. The civilisation in which we live today, in the electronic and information age, seems already to have reached a peak, from where it can only go downhill. Already there is a visible deterioration in our way of life. Our values, both moral and material, are changing rapidly and humanity's indifference to and exploitation of nature and the world's environment can only lead us on a path towards disaster.

THE WRONG KIND OF FOOD

Did you realise that during the past 100 to 150 years eating habits in Western industrialised countries have changed more than in the previous 5,000 to 6,000 years?

Food which at one time was very expensive became cheaper, and at last most people could afford to buy meat, fruit and sweets and eat their fill. Today in Europe and the USA we live in a time of abundance never before known; in fact, in this part of the world there is more food available than people need. But are we any healthier because of this? No – quite the contrary! Never before in history have so many people been chronically ill. The food we eat today no longer contains the necessary nutrients needed for the correct functioning of our digestive system, and therefore most of our diseases are caused by, and start with, metabolic disorders.

Due to the over-consumption of de-natured food, and a lack of exercise and fresh air, many people, especially in the second half of their lives, often become caricatures of themselves. There is not much left of the Grecian ideal of a beautiful human being. Nowadays we rarely see a really beautiful and healthy-looking person. Most of us are comfort-loving gourmets or gourmands and we are either too fat or too thin. Our legs are swollen, our feet flat, our backs bent, our necks stiff. We lose our hair, suffer from dental decay, headaches, flatulence, constipation and depression; we tire quickly and, worst of all, many of us no longer enjoy life. Many people never feel really well.

An Austrian newspaper, *Das Kurier*, dated 15 May, 1997, stated: 'More and more young people enjoy poor health. Over two million Austrians feel physically impaired. This tendency among young people is increasing. About 30 per cent of all Austrians are physically affected in their daily lives.' This shows that even the younger generation is not as healthy as in the past. Austria is not the only country with such problems. More and more people in our industrialised countries suffer from chronic diseases, and others who think they are healthy should take another look at their health. Nowadays people seem to think that dental decay, headaches, allergies and other such ailments are normal and that one 'just has to live' with these problems. This idea is nonsense!

Health problems always have a reason. When the human organism goes on strike and does not function correctly, there must be a cause for it. Our organism is a kind of living machine, which, like any other machine, needs a specific type of fuel. Apart from oxygen and water, our most important fuel is our nutrition. Before we were born, our body was built with the help of this fuel. Therefore, it is very important that a future mother should eat healthy food, as this builds up the fundamental framework of the body and mind of her child.

The foundation of any building must be firm and should be built only with top quality materials. Likewise, a healthy body can be built and maintained only with first class food. All other factors, even if they seem to be elemental, are of secondary importance. No disease can be healed, even with the best medicine, if one does not eat a healthy diet.

Gᴇɴᴇᴛɪᴄ Fᴀᴄᴛᴏʀs

And what about genes? Genes certainly make up the foundations of the body. As long as the person concerned maintains a healthy lifestyle and eats the right food, if there are no extremely harmful influences, most negative genetic factors remain latent (dormant) and will not cause any damage. In a healthy organism, viruses, bacteria and other micro-organisms can seldom multiply unrestrainedly. The defence system of a healthy body does not allow this to happen.

Iɴᴅᴜsᴛʀɪᴀʟ ᴀᴅᴜʟᴛᴇʀᴀᴛɪᴏɴ ᴏꜰ ᴏᴜʀ ꜰᴏᴏᴅ

As I explained before, our organism adapted itself to the life and the eating habits of the first primitive people during its original evolution. Since then and as long as human nutrition did not change too much, the assimilation, the transformation and the utilisation of food was never much of a problem for our digestive organs. However, in the course of time human nutritional habits changed in many ways. There were migrations of people to other continents, where the food was completely different. Sometimes it was difficult and took quite some time for their digestive organs to adapt to a new kind of nutrition. But as the food was still completely natural and contained most of the nutrients the human body needed, the organism, after some time, adjusted itself quite well.

Unfortunately, during the last 100 to 150 years the situation has changed increasingly in the negative sense. Now the chances of the survival of the human race are not threatened primarily by nuclear danger, but by the degeneration and chronic diseases caused mainly by the malnutrition from which the inhabitants of industrialised countries suffer. Many of the foods we eat today are completely incompatible with our digestive systems.

For our body the assimilation and transformation of this so-called 'food' is extremely difficult. While in prehistoric times all food was 100 per cent natural, today 80 per cent of our modern food has been adulterated to such an extent that it contains hardly any vitamins, minerals or other vital substances. It does, however, contain calories!

Our food still contains proteins, carbohydrates and fats, which unfortunately have been modified in many ways. Most of this food has been over-heated, pressed, cooled, tumbled, frozen or defrosted, and during every one of these procedures vital nutrients are lost and countless additives are used to replace them.

New foods are invented all the time; many colourings and uncountable substances are used to enhance the taste and appearance of the food. The consumer often has no idea what he or she is actually eating. During the process of refining our food, manufacturers use up to 3,500 mostly chemical additives. Quite a few of these additives may be harmful or even poisonous for the human organism, but as long as this has not been proved absolutely the food can still be sold. Most people believe that the quantities of these substances used for the 'refining' of our food are so small that they can do no harm. Also, those responsible for our health do not seem to know that many such substances could have a toxic or even lethal effect, even when diluted a hundred or a thousand times. Of course, the defence mechanisms of our bodies are able to render many of these toxins harmless. However, any person who, over a long period of time, consumes often the same foods or soft drinks will finally accumulate so many harmful substances in his body that he or she will no longer be able to eliminate them.

Fast food and modern drinks

During the last century, we seem to have forgotten which foods are really suitable for us. Children eat sweets and drink cola drinks and parents wonder why their little darlings are so restless or look so pale.

Not only the body but also the nervous system and the brain are receiving artificial substitutes instead of the needed nutrients. So-called fast food and ready-made meals, which are absolutely useless for our health, have become bestsellers. We have less work to do in the kitchen; we only have to add a little water to some of these dishes and put them in the microwave oven, and they are ready to eat. Soup, gravies and sauces often contain nothing but salt, flavourings and other chemical ingredients which never deserve to be called natural. We are so used to products such as potato-chips, crisps and all kinds of other snacks that we no longer think of them as harmful. We are used to this kind of food, but our organism will never get used to it!

As all or most of the vital nutrients in food are destroyed, manufacturers often add minute quantities of synthetic vitamins and minerals. Although insignificant, these quantities may then be printed on the label along with the other ingredients. This is pure fraud! One cannot take away almost all of the valuable nutrients and then replace part of them by with artificially made substances. The chemical formula is correct, but these substances can never be compared with natural vitamins and minerals. They lack vitality and life, which cannot be reproduced in a factory.

Modern drinks are just as bad or even worse. In former days people drank only water, or sometimes, as an exception, a little beer or wine which was diluted with water. When very thirsty, people drank water mixed with a little vinegar. In modern society people drink more and more alcohol and this tendency continues to rise. Many children and adults drink soft drinks instead of water. The consumption of these drinks is estimated as being on average 130 litres per person annually. In North America this figure is even higher. Most of these drinks contain an excess of sugar and additives, as well as many calories, which spoil a healthy appetite. Many people have developed an addiction to coffee and cola drinks. These problems will be discussed in detail later in this book.

What is meant by 'living food'?

The major part of our modern food has become, as Professor Kollath often said, 'lifeless food'. It has been killed by different manipulations, and can no longer sustain its metabolic activity. The best example is a grain of cereal. As I already pointed out, grains will not spoil for thousands of years if they are stored correctly. Grains which were found in Egyptian tombs can still germinate today, if they are planted in good soil. They still contain enzymes and other vital ingredients, which are needed for our own growth and health.

A cereal grain is composed of the following parts: the husk, the flower and the seed. The smallest part is the seed, which guarantees the propagation of the cereal species. Although its weight is only 10 per cent of the entire grain, the seed contains all the enzymes and other nutrients. However, because of all these enzymes the seed tastes a little bitter and for commercial purposes this is a disadvantage. It also becomes rancid very quickly and so not only the husk but also the seed is discarded during the process of grinding. The husks and seeds are then sold as high-quality animal feed. What is left is the flour, which contains only calories and hardly any essential nutrients. As in the case of most other industrialised food, living food has been turned into a dead product and the animals get the better deal.

When, in the year 1900, the well-known Swiss

physician Max Bircher-Benner spoke to an audience of physicians in Zurich, Switzerland, nobody seemed to understand quite what he meant when he spoke about the dynamic healing power of raw food and vegetables. They were not able to understand that raw vegetables contain very special nutrients which no longer exist when cooked. The general comment after his lecture was that: 'Dr Bircher has gone beyond the borders of science.' But as his special diet became more and more successful, there were many intelligent physicians who became interested in his therapy. In his clinic in Zurich, Dr Bircher-Benner treated not only Swiss patients, but also many patients from the USA, Australia and even Japan with raw vegetables, fruit and his famous breakfast food, 'Bircher-muesli'. This is similar to our 'granola'. Further research has largely confirmed his ideas.

HANS-PETER RUSCH

In the year 1949 Dr Hans-Peter Rusch wrote in his work on *The Circulation of Living Substances* that in everything alive there must be tiny 'living units', which transfer 'life from one being to another'.

We receive our most important source of energy from the rays of the sun, not only directly but also indirectly, through our food. In order to understand this, we must first of all look at the soil. A healthy soil contains many substances which plants need for their growth and development, such as nitrogen, potassium, phosphorus, chalk etc. In order to absorb all these nutrients from the soil, the plant needs help. The micro-flora in the soil consists of an army of millions of bacteria, fungi and other micro-organisms which help plants to absorb all these nutrients and eliminate waste. Alongside this micro-flora there is also the macro-flora, whose task it is to digest the soil and keep it loose. Earthworms, moles and insects, among others, belong to this group of macro-flora. This living community in the soil, the micro- and macro-flora, should always be well balanced. Only when this flora is healthy and not interfered with is it possible for the plants to absorb their nutrients from the soil and produce important and essential vital nutrients for human beings and animals.

Plants are able, with the help of a green pigment from their leaves, and under the influence of sunlight, to create carbohydrates, fats, proteins and other vital substances. If, with our modern agricultural methods, we destroy the micro- and macro-flora instead of improving the soil, the plants can no longer absorb all the nutrients they need. By using artificial fertilisers, on the one hand the essential requirements of the plants are ignored and on the other hand they get far too much of certain substances such as nitrogen. Thus, the soil is destroyed to such a degree that the plants living in it contain only a small fraction of their former nutritional value.

Many plants become weak and diseased and are then treated with chemical 'healing remedies', just like human beings. In this way the micro- and macro-flora are destroyed more and more, until the soil becomes a dead substance. A similar thing happens to people who are continually treated with antibiotics or other chemical substances. In the human body, as well as in the soil, bacteria play a vital part in all processes. Our body contains more bacteria than cells, all of which have their special functions. Only a very small percentage of these bacteria can be classified as harmful *or even dangerous*.

The energy of the sun

The well-known physical chemist Wilhelm Oswald stated many years ago: 'When we eat plants, we eat energy coming from the sun'. At that time this was only a theory, but today we know it to be true.'

By electro-magnetic measuring methods, physical and electro-chemical investigations and many other methods, one can now prove many facts, which were, at the beginning of the 20th century, based only upon the well-thought-out hypotheses of some courageous scientists and physicians.

CHAPTER TWO

Digestion

Normal and abnormal digestion

According to their digestive organs and their teeth, human beings belong to the category of 'fructivores' (fruit eaters). This does not mean that humans should live exclusively on fruit, but it does show that by nature they are best suited to eat cereals, roots, fruit, nuts and many other products of the soil. This does not exclude them from eating animal products once in a while. One must understand, however, that for us animal protein is basically a 'second-hand' food, as most of the energy an animal receives from plant food has already been used by its own body.

In the previous chapter I pointed out that only about 20 per cent of our modern food remains natural. We eat far too much animal protein, refined carbohydrates and the wrong kind of fat. We eat too much, too fast, too often and usually at the wrong time of the day. In the following chapters I will show you how well a healthy body functions when given the right kind of food, and also why we become ill when we eat things which cannot, or can only partly, be metabolised in the human body.

Unsuitable nutrition is one of the most important causes of all our civilisation's diseases and of our disastrous state of health. The second cause is the wrong kind of medical treatment. This will be explained in all possible detail in the three volumes of this series.

THE DIGESTION OF FOOD IN THE MOUTH

The normal process
As food in former times was hard, rough, tough and fibrous, people had to chew it thoroughly for a long time. All carbohydrates from bread, cereals, potatoes, rice etc. were broken up by enzymes in the saliva and thus prepared for digestion in the stomach and the intestines. The food was mixed with up to 1.5 litres of saliva each day and specific antibodies in the mouth ensured that innumerable bacteria and toxins were destroyed there. The chewing also stimulated the blood circulation of the gums and dental decay was rare.

The abnormal process
As our modern food is soft and contains very little fibre, we no longer have to chew so thoroughly. Many things are swallowed before being saturated with saliva and thus part of the carbohydrate in the food cannot be broken up. Every year more additives and other artificial substances find their way into food, and the antibodies in the mouth are unable to detoxify such quantities.

Many toxins then pass into the throat, where the defence mechanism of the tonsils cannot always cope with so much work. They become enlarged and inflamed, causing difficulty in breathing. How many children one sees today with their mouths agape, not due to lack of intelligence, but mainly because the defence mechanism of their lymphatic systems, which includes the tonsils, is continually overstrained through an over-consumption of dairy produce, sweets and soft drinks. Up to a few years ago the tonsils were often removed when they became inflamed, but the medical fraternity has now learned that they fulfill important tasks in the human body and that their removal provides only temporary help. The cause of the swelling and inflammation is not eliminated, and the side effects, such as bronchitis, asthma and sinus problems, still remain. The only remedy lies in an immediate change of diet and intensive natural treatment.

As people no longer chew properly, dentists only exceptionally see gums which receive a fresh blood supply. The roots of the teeth are undernourished and gradually become loose. When the body lacks certain minerals and other nutrients, its most important task is to make sure that the essential organs receive all the vital nutrients available. The survival of the entire organism depends upon this. Teeth and bones are not essential and therefore, in an emergency, the needed minerals are removed from the easily dissolved mineral deposits of the bones and the teeth. Thus, one can understand that tooth decay is not only a local problem, but a sign of a general complicated disturbance of the entire organism. Not only elderly people but even babies and small children can suffer from a lack of minerals and from a degeneration of the jawbones.

As a result of modern malnutrition, the composition of the saliva changes and bacteria thrive through constant contact with sugar and sweets. The waste products of these bacteria in the mouth cause a hyper-acidity and this acid attacks the dental enamel. Most of our modern food is far too acidic and in the long run all of these different kinds of acid will destroy our teeth. Not only things which taste acidic, but also any kind of sugar or sweets provoke an acid reaction in our digestive tracts.

You can prove to yourself quite easily that acids can destroy your teeth. In order to do a test, put some vinegar or lemon juice into a little jar and then put a little bone or a tooth into the jar and close. If, after some weeks you open the jar again, you will find that the little bone, or the tooth, are not there anymore; they have been dissolved by the acid. So, please be aware of acids and sweets!

Factors like malnutrition, acidity and bacteria interact and caries, tartar and pyorrhea develop. These problems cannot be prevented, even by intensive brushing of the teeth, particularly as the consumption of sugar and sweets increases each year. But, after all, the food industry should also be allowed to do business! Sooner or later the teeth begin to fall out and people need dentures. It seems that already 90 per cent of all children going to school have caries.

Albrecht von Haller, in *Gefährdete Menschheit* (*Endangered Humanity*), could already prove many years ago that primitive people who start eating white flour, sugar and sweets will, within a few years, show deficiency symptoms which start with tooth decay.

THE DIGESTION IN THE STOMACH

The normal process
Food will be liquidised in the mouth, thereby breaking up all the carbohydrates into different parts which will then pass through the gullet (esophagus) into the stomach. Gastric juices, which are alkaline in the mouth, become acid in the stomach, where the nutrient solution is kneaded for a long time by the contractions of the stomach wall. At the same time, the transformation of starches into sugar takes place, special enzymes digest all the proteins from the food and the stomach acid kills the remaining harmful bacteria and neutralises toxic substances.

The stomach wall is covered by a layer of mucus, which is renewed constantly and therefore cannot be attacked by the gastric acid. Depending on the kind of food, the nutrient solution remains between one and eight hours in the stomach. When the digestion has been completed, the contents of the stomach will slowly be emptied into the upper part of the small intestine, namely the duodenum.

The abnormal process
When the nutrients have not been sufficiently liquidised in the mouth, part of the carbohydrates cannot be broken up. These nutrients then enter the stomach, where a more intensive digestion is needed. This nutrient solution contains many highly concentrated substances, such as sugar, white flour or fruit juices. For such highly concentrated foods there are no adequate digestive juices available. Glands which could produce such juices would have to be developed first. For this reason it may still take

a very long time before human beings are able to digest such refined foods without problems.

Nevertheless, the stomach does make an effort to digest these concentrates and provides huge quantities of normal digestive juices for this alien food. As only very little of these juices will actually be used the rest remain in the stomach, with the risk that these very acidic juices will irritate and eventually destroy part of the stomach wall. In order to prevent this, and to protect the stomach wall, the organism will begin to produce vast quantities of mucus. However, a stomach filled with mucus cannot digest food properly and the nutrient solution stays far too long in the stomach, where it begins to ferment and produces much gas. People suffer from wind and a tight feeling in their abdomen. Sometimes, if animal protein and starches are eaten at the same time, because of too much acidity the transformation of starches cannot take place. However, this always depends on the different quantities of animal protein and starches eaten during a meal. Because of this, many of my patients follow the advice given in *Fit for Life* by Les Snowdon and Maggie Humphreys and similar health books, and try not to eat starches and animal protein at the same meal.

THE DIGESTION IN THE SMALL INTESTINE

The normal process
After the nutrient solution has been digested in the stomach it is slowly passed on into the duodenum, where it is mixed with the gastric juices secreted by the pancreas and the gall bladder. The bile from the gall bladder breaks

up fats, which are then transported via the lymph glands to the liver. The juices of the pancreas are alkaline and neutralise the nutrient solution after it has left the very acidic milieu of the stomach. The nutrient solution is then pushed further into the small intestine, where the digestion becomes more intensive.

The intestines are moving constantly in order to mix the nutrient solution with the gastric juices. About five hours later the digestion in the small intestine has been completed. Gradually the various food components are assimilated and filtered by small filters located in the wall of the intestines. The nutrients are then passed into a net of tiny blood vessels (capillaries) located in and behind the intestinal wall. The filtered blood from all these tiny vessels then flows into a much larger blood vessel, the vena porta, and from there it goes into the liver, where it is cleansed once again.

The abnormal process
The partly digested nutrient solution is slowly pushed from the stomach into the duodenum. However, when gas pressure builds up because of huge quantities of mucus, the entire stomach contents may suddenly be emptied into the duodenum. When the latter happens, the gastric juices of the intestines can no longer neutralise all the acid of the nutrient solution quickly enough and the acid then attacks the intestinal wall. Thus, inflammation or even ulcers can develop.

Nowadays, I see in my daily practice more and more people suffering from gastric and intestinal diseases. Most people do not realise that such diseases could easily have been prevented, and that is a great pity. The food we eat cannot be used by our bodies unless it has been broken down into its basic substances and changed into 'endogen' substances. Only these substances can be assimilated and digested, and will then pass into our blood through the filters in the intestinal wall.

If this pressure builds up, the entire stomach contents may suddenly be emptied into the duodenum. In this case the nutrient solution is very acid and results in the intestines becoming irritated. This can be the cause of ulcers. Nowadays more and more people suffer from gastric and intestinal diseases.

What about snacks between meals?
Not long ago, doctors used to think it healthier to eat small quantities of food several times during the day instead of large meals. This would make the digestion of food easier. This idea is not altogether wrong, as nobody should eat too much food at one time. However, it has now been proved that even for diabetics eating between meals is basically wrong, as the following happens.

As soon as the nutrient solution reaches the stomach, digestion begins. This process, depending upon the kind of food eaten, takes an average of four to five hours. After this food has been digested in the stomach it will slowly be passed into the duodenum. If at such a moment new, undigested food comes into the stomach, it will be passed directly into the upper intestines, together with the already digested food, and will be the cause of many health problems. In that case, only the already digested nutrients can pass through the very small filters of the intestinal wall. The rest stays in the small intestine much too long and begins to ferment.

Although a certain amount of fermentation is completely normal, semi-digested food causing super-fermentation in the upper part of the intestines can then, because of air pressure, be pushed into the large intestine or even lower. This can cause much gas, pain and inflammation. It is therefore better not to eat between meals, except perhaps some fruit once in a while, which will be quickly digested.

It is the task of the small intestine to break up the food into its basic substances, such as carbohydrates, proteins, fats, vitamins, minerals etc. Because of our modern eating habits, this task has become very difficult. The nutrient solution often contains molecules which can only be digested with much effort, and there are always more concentrated and unnatural substances.

The residual toxins and irritating substances, in the long run, damage the sensitive intestinal wall and the small filters which it contains become either clogged or porous. In this way more and more useless substances end up in the capillaries or in the surrounding tissues. The rest of the nutrient solution (undigested food, fibres, chemicals and other unnatural substances) is now pushed into the bowels by alternating contractions and relaxation of the ring muscles of the bowels.

Bottlenecks in the intestines
The muscular movements of the intestines are controlled by hormones and triggered off by neural impulses. If, however, the food contains too little fibre, the nervous net in the intestinal wall will not be sufficiently stimulated, the bowel movements slow down and the continuous supply of food causes blockages in the intestinal loops (bends). The food residue remains too long in these bends; it

ferments, turns bad, becomes dry and hardens. In these areas inflammation can easily develop. It may take years until the person who suffers from such an inflammation realises this, because the feeling of pain in the abdomen is very slight.

Very few people in our Western countries who are over 50 have normally shaped intestines. If the pressure in the intestines augments because of blockages or gas, their shape changes. They distend in certain areas, lose their elasticity and become flabby; in other areas they contract, become thinner and cramped. Often their location also changes and some parts of the intestines and the bowels shift to areas where they do not belong. The digestive organs lose their support and this allows them to be displaced. This again results in their malfunction; the abdomen becomes bloated and loses its once-juvenile shape.

THE DIGESTION IN THE LARGE INTESTINE

The normal process
After all the nutrients are assimilated into the blood, the fibres and further residual substances of the nutrient solution pass into the large intestine. There, billions of bacteria accomplish important tasks. They live on the fibres, from which they extract the last nutrients. These bacteria are very important for us; they produce vitamins, especially those of the B-group, and help to eliminate harmful substances and germs. They have many more functions about which, at this time, we still know very little.

Also in the large intestine, the nutrient solution is pushed further down by the movements of the ring muscles of the intestinal wall. The more fibres there are, the more the nerves in the intestinal wall will be stimulated and the sooner the excrement, by way of the bowels, can be disposed of. Sometimes this process can be influenced by psychological problems, but on the whole the composition of the daily food is the most important factor by which to prevent hard excrement.

The nutrient solution, which was very liquid in the small intestine, loses more and more fluid during its passage through the large intestine. The further the nutrient solution travels into the lower sections of the bowels, the more compact it becomes. Fibrous substances play an important part here. They are able to retain a lot of water and at the same time they see to it that the excrement does not become too dry. Good excrement still contains about 70 per cent of water and is not sticky.

Dr Dennis Burkitt, an Irish physician and scientist, world-famous for his books and publications on the value of fibre in our food, examined the eating habits of African tribes in the year 1971. He compared these with the eating habits of Europeans and discovered that the tribes ate much fibrous food, which passed through their intestines in less than 30 hours, the weight of the excrement being between 300 and 500 grams. An Englishman's excrement weighed between 80 and 120 grams, and the average time it took to pass through the intestines was 70 hours. Burkitt believed that many of our Western diseases, from which the Africans suffer only exceptionally, are caused mainly by a lack of fibre in the diet.

The excrement of a healthy person contains only a small

quantity of food at the end of its journey through the large intestine and the colon, or even no food at all. It contains mainly bacteria, skin flakes and useless substances.

The abnormal process
If we always ate food which was appropriate for our digestive system, we would – as you have seen – digest everything without any problem. When, however, we eat food which is unsuitable for our organism, exactly the opposite happens. Day by day we make so many nutritional errors that it is hard to say which is the worst. Doubtless a combination of different mistakes, continually made, is the most important cause of our so-called 'civilisation diseases'.

While describing abnormal digestive processes, I mentioned how, through a sudden gas pressure, the nutrient solution can get into the lower sections of the intestines. The upper part of the small intestine is practically sterile, but further down there are innumerable bacteria that live exclusively on fibre and food residues. These different strains of bacteria are very useful to us and they normally remain in balance, meaning that none of these strains can multiply in such a way as to be dangerous to our health. When, however, there is suddenly an abundance of undigested food, this balance is disturbed in favour of harmful bacteria, which then have a real feast. These 'putrefactive' bacteria multiply very fast, and their metabolic waste (excrement) causes the formation of gas and dangerous toxins like indol and scatol. The person in question feels bloated and gets a stomach-ache, and his abdomen swells.

The immune system of the large intestine is thus

continually overstrained and alien substances, toxins or harmful bacteria enter the body tissues. As a result of the irritant effect of these substances, there is the possibility of inflammation in any part of the body. A typical example is ulcers of the anus, which are more commonplace than one would think possible in our time. Another problem is the ever-increasing fungal diseases. Fungi can only multiply unchecked when most of the enteric bacteria (gut-friendly bacteria) have been destroyed by antibiotics, or in some other way. The consumption of refined carbohydrates supports the growth of fungi, as they prefer to live on sugar, like many other small creatures. A fungal infection can spread to any part of the body and cause dangerous diseases. More and more people die from fungal infections.

BOWEL PROBLEMS

In the Western world 40–50 per cent of the population suffers temporarily, sometimes chronically, from constipation. For women the percentage is even higher, around 70 per cent. If the food is lacking in fibre, the nerve net, which surrounds the large intestine, is not sufficiently stimulated. In this case the nutrient solution often remains for days, sometimes even for weeks, in the intestines, slowly becoming drier and drier. It is very possible that the person in question still goes once in a while to the toilet or even has diarrhoea, but even then part of the excrement will keep sticking to the bowels. Fermenting excrement and other toxins create a very poisonous environment, which can cause serious diseases, like colitis ulcerosa, diverticulosis or Crohn's disease. There is also the risk of a re-intoxication in the upper intestinal regions. The root of many diseases is located in the intestines.

One of the most important tasks of the large intestine is to withdraw water from the nutrient solution so that the excrement in the colon will have the right consistency. Fibre normally keeps the excrement soft. If this is missing, constipation can easily develop. Coffee, black tea, cola and other soft drinks are dehydrating and worsen these problems in the long run. These drinks also irritate the kidneys, thereby withdrawing fluid from the water supply of the body.

THE INFLUENCE OF THE INTESTINES ON POSTURE AND BACK PROBLEMS (A HYPOTHESIS OF DR KARL-OTTO HEEDE)

Few people suspect that, for example, scoliosis, a curvature of the spine, spondylosis, back pain, lumbago and other back problems are often related to the condition of our digestive organs. A normal posture has become rare, and changes in the form of the thoracic cage (chest) are often the consequences of diseases of the abdomen, shifting of the organs and, above all, of a constant pressure of gas in the abdominal cavity.

Without our being aware of it, this can release enormous forces, especially when this pressure always occurs in the same parts of the body. In that case, first of all some vertebrae of the chest will be pressed slowly outwards, so that in the course of some years the youthful waistline will disappear, a phenomenon which can be observed with most elderly people. In the case of a strong formation of gas in the abdominal cavity, any weak vertebrae, as well as the bones of the neck and the spine, can become dislocated or deformed. Even when people are still young there can be a deviation of the spine because of this. Always, the organism will try to compensate for this by taking counter-measures, by drawing in part of the spine or by exerting a counter pressure on the corresponding vertebrae in the spine. Consequently, lordosis, a hollow back, can develop as well as spondylosis, scoliosis and other serious problems which can sometimes be very painful. Doctors try to cure these problems by using physiotherapy, bath treatments, gymnastics, chiropractic therapy, massage and different drugs; sometimes with, and sometimes without success. When the abdominal cavity has not been thoroughly examined and the often diseased intestines have not been treated, the physician can at best expect a temporary improvement, but nothing more.

Such treatments can take years, often many years, and all of them are insufficient if all the causes are not recognised and eliminated. Besides all these, in themselves excellent treatments, the most important thing would be to treat the original causes as well.

Dr Bircher-Benner was very successful when treating patients who suffered from rheumatic diseases and problems of the spine by prescribing the right kind of diet. The wrong kind of nutrition, and food, which is lacking in many vital substances, weakens the muscles, the bones, the vertebrae and the spine.

The worst offenders
The following substances are mainly responsible for the shocking state of our health:

◆ refined carbohydrates, such as sugar and refined flour
◆ refined fats
◆ food additives
◆ chemical residues from agriculture and stock breeding
◆ chemical and synthetic drugs
◆ addictive and unsuitable drinks

There is a clear connection between the intensive mechanical and chemical denaturalisation of our food and the typical diseases of our modern time. Every era has had its specific diseases, which were caused by the special conditions of that time. They depended on social, religious, economic, climatic and other environmental influences, as well as on the emotional lives of people during that period. Nutritional habits and the kind of foods we eat are largely influenced by these elemental facts. Bad nutritional habits and an inadequate and unbalanced diet, combined with other factors, were always the basis upon which diseases could develop.

Since prehistoric times the type and composition of the food we eat has often changed, and people have always been able to adapt to these changes. When nothing else is available man can live mainly on carbohydrates or animal protein for a long time, and he can survive on very little food. However, the ability of man to adapt is not unlimited. When natural food is treated ever more intensively and all the special ingredients which we need for our survival are removed, when natural products are turned into artificial products, which have nothing in common with the original food, people cannot stay healthy. Therefore, on the following pages I will describe in greater detail what effects the worst offenders have on our health.

REFINED CARBOHYDRATES

Sugar

Sometimes health fanatics will tell you: 'Sugar is poison.' However, there is no need to regard sugar in quite such an extreme way. Sugar only becomes a problem when refined industrialised sugar is used regularly and unfortunately most people do this, often without realising it. This is because the sugar you eat comes not only from the sugar bowl but is also hidden in all kinds of food, even where you would never expect it to be.

Food manufacturers love to use sugar. In the first place, sugar is one of the best ways in which to preserve all kinds of food, as bacteria cannot live on such a highly concentrated substance. In the second place, they love to use sugar because it is addictive, and everything prepared with some sugar sells extremely well. In former times, the sugar people consumed came from fruit, vegetables, tubers or roots. Honey was a rarity. In the 15th century, in tropical countries, sugar was extracted from sugar cane and exported in small quantities to Europe; however, it was extremely expensive. Then, about 200 years ago, people learned to extract sugar from sugar beets. In the beginning, this procedure was very difficult and expensive and for a long time sugar still remained a luxury. Today everyone can afford to buy cheap, refined sugar, which is totally different from the natural product. Through extraction, heating, bleaching etc, the manufacturers have produced an artificial, concentrated substance which contains hardly any of the vital substances we need, only calories. Sugar has been turned into a lifeless substance, which will damage our health if consumed regularly. This applies to any kind of sugar, perhaps with the exception of small quantities of natural honey or natural cane sugar, provided that both products have been treated in the old manner and have not been adulterated in any way. However, even of those only minimal quantities are recommended, as such natural products are very concentrated.

Sugar is a vitamin and mineral thief
When sugar is manufactured, all the fibres, vitamins and minerals contained in the original product are discarded. However, the human organism cannot metabolise sugar or any other refined food when these vital substances are missing. Therefore minerals and other vital substances have to be confiscated from the body's own reserves, which can be found, for example, in our teeth and bones. Even small children who eat many sweets and pastries, then, will suffer from dental decay.

For the same reason many elderly people lose their teeth and, because of lack of exercise and bad eating habits, their bones become brittle and weak. Although nowadays in many homes for the elderly they serve a raw salad with or before the meal, coffee, a sweet dessert or a pastry is highly appreciated. This is a very bad custom, because refined sugar or flour in combination with raw salads will cause much fermentation in the intestines, a stomach-ache, flatulence and even more serious health problems.

The more sugar we eat the greater becomes our lack of B vitamins, which are extremely important for our nerves.

Nervous people and restless, sleepless children love sweets!

The blood sugar level and the addiction to sugar
While in a healthy body the metabolism of sugar from fruit, raw vegetables and cereals, which still contain all their original vital substances (vitamins, minerals etc.), is never problematic, concentrated refined carbohydrates can be the cause of a sudden steep rise of the blood sugar level, called hyperglycaemia.

The pancreas produces insulin, needed for the assimilation of sugar. However, in the case of refined sugar the pancreas produces far too much insulin. In nature sugar always is combined with fibre, vitamins, minerals and other substances, so our pancreas still produces the quantity of insulin needed for the digestion of sugar cane or big sugar beets, instead of producing only the insulin needed for a small amount of sugar. After this sugar has been 'digested', there is still much insulin available, which should be used in some way. Now the craving for something sweet starts, and at the same time the blood sugar level in the blood drops lower and lower. This condition is called hypoglycaemia and may cause extreme weakness, dizziness, fainting or even circulatory failure.

The person affected thus will often go out of their way to obtain something sweet. As soon as, for example, they eat some chocolate, the craving abates, the level of the blood sugar goes up and everything is fine until the now-available sugar in its turn has been used. This can go on and on, and in this way a real addiction to sweets develops, which can be the cause of many serious diseases.

This again shows that any natural food which has been

industrially manipulated and disorganised has become an alien substance to the human body. It can disrupt normally well-balanced digestive processes, and cause functional disorders and many different diseases.

Wholemeal flour versus refined flour

All refined carbohydrates, such as sugar and refined flour, with the exception of freshly ground wholemeal flour, lack vitamins, minerals and other vital substances. These vital substances which are missing in such refined products are confiscated from the body's own supplies. If refined flour is combined with sugar, the body is deprived of still more vital nutrients.

For thousands of years, cereals were the staple food of most people. Cereal grains contain practically all the nutrients we need in order to be healthy. However, modern food technology manages to alter this and to manufacture completely useless products, which not only are the cause of obesity but also, amongst other problems, of constipation, from which more than 50 per cent of the Western world suffers.

Because our modern food contains ever-decreasing amounts of vital substances, sooner or later the body's defences weaken. The acidity which occurs in the organism when there is a lack of vital substances helps to produce all kinds of infections and the 'diseases of civilisation'. B vitamins, which are lost during the refining of food, play an important role in the digestion of carbohydrates. When carbohydrates, due to this lack, cannot be completely digested, toxic substances accumulate in the body tissues and this can be the prerequisite for the development of malignant cells. The WHO (World Health Organisation) expects an enormous increase in several types of cancer in the next ten to 20 years.

These B vitamins are also most important for the nervous system and the brain. People who eat many refined carbohydrates, especially children, are often extremely nervous. Also, mental illness, and Alzheimer's disease, is on the increase in all industrial countries.

WHAT ABOUT FAT?

Not so long ago, fat was a scarce commodity and was highly appreciated. Nowadays, everybody knows that we eat far too much fat. In North America the 'anti-fat-movement' is an exaggerated reaction to the great problems with which the many obese people in that country have to cope. Research shows that 40 per cent of the American diet consists of fat, and now many Americans have a 'fat phobia'; they do not dare to eat the slightest amount of fat. This means good business for the food industry and every supermarket and grocery store has started selling low-fat products, which they advertise in capital letters.

The average American citizen and many doctors are convinced that health problems such as obesity, heart and circulatory diseases etc. are caused almost exclusively by the consumption of too much fat. This simply is not true! In believing this, one overlooks the important fact that sugar and other refined products, for example, are just as much to blame for the development of these diseases.

It is wrong and even dangerous to exclude every kind of

fat from our nutrition – we need fat! Fats give us warmth and muscle power. Essential fatty acids are vital for the structure of our body cells and for their perfect function. Some vitamins cannot be utilised without fat. Fat has many important functions in our body.

Different kinds of fat
We do need fat, but not just any kind of fat. Some fats are good for us, but some are bad for our health. The best fats are the natural unsaturated and polyunsaturated fats, which we find in natural foods like avocados, nuts and natural oils, which have not been treated industrially or changed in any way. However, as soon as these unsaturated fats are heated they become saturated.

Natural unsaturated fats are, because of their biochemical structure, able to combine with natural proteins and thus play an important role in the transportation and utilization of oxygen in our body. Such fats are easy to digest, whereas saturated fats can have the same kind of destructive effect on all organic functions as dangerous poisons. They damage the red blood corpuscles as well as the composition of the blood and, in combination with too much protein, they cause many chronic diseases such as diabetes, arteriosclerosis, cirrhosis of the liver and thrombosis.

Because of our polluted environment we find, mainly in animal fat, highly poisonous fat-soluble chemicals, such as insecticides, herbicides, detergents etc. These harmful animal fats, as well as synthetic fats, impair oxygen utilization and respiratory processes, which are extremely important for a healthy metabolism. Among the animal fats we can recommend only butter, as almost all kinds of margarine are lifeless industrial products, and hardly ever contain healthy unsaturated fats. Butter contains many substances which are absolutely vital to our health. If once in a while you eat meat which contains some fat, it will not kill you. However, do not make a habit of this.

On the other hand, an avocado pear contains the right kind of fat and you certainly will not gain any weight when you eat half an avocado, with some lemon juice and not with mayonnaise. These natural unsaturated oils lower the cholesterol content in the blood, prevent blood corpuscles from sticking together and lower the blood pressure. They help fight infections, prevent thrombosis and liver damage, and also have a soothing effect on the nervous system. Nervous, hyperactive children should regularly take some unsaturated oil – about 2–3 teaspoons daily.

You will find good unsaturated oils mainly in health food shops, and you should always keep these oils in the refrigerator as otherwise they soon become rancid. Vitamin C, magnesium, vitamin B and, above all, zinc are needed for the easy digestion of the healthy fat you need.

FOOD ADDITIVES

Until around 100–150 years ago, only natural ways and means of preserving food were known. Food was dried in the sun, in the air or at the fireplace, or was preserved by the use of sugar, salty or sour liquids, oil or starches. Later, preservation was achieved through heat and eventually by using very low temperatures or ice.

When fruit and vegetables, for example, have not been changed by mechanical or chemical methods, freezing and drying are still the best and healthiest ways of preserving food. However, as soon as fresh, natural food has been processed and adulterated by industrial manipulations in order to become non-perishable, it becomes a low-quality food which has lost all, or at least a great part, of its vital ingredients. Although some of these products still contain proteins, carbohydrates and fats, these have generally been changed to such an extent that they become worthless, harmful or even dangerous for our health when we eat them regularly. The preserving of food has become a very important commercial factor. About 80 per cent of all food in supermarkets today is either tinned, or food which has been treated in many different ways in order to increase its shelf life or to improve its appearance.

While a natural product is being processed it loses its attractive appearance, its taste and its smell. Today this is not a problem any longer. The chemical industry offers many substances which will enhance the taste and the smell of anything, and can change even the most appalling looking and smelling food into a gourmet dream which says 'Buy me!' In 1950, about 700 such additives were already officially permitted. Today there are over 4,000 additives available which contain hardly any natural ingredients.

It is such a pity that our organism does not produce any digestive juices which can digest additives! Many additives used for food preserving can paralyse or even kill bacteria or other very small creatures which happen to be in the food. People do not seem to know that bacteria and human cells are very similar; both of them have their own metabolisms and are highly sensitive to strong toxins. We may assume that such additives in our bodies would have a similar effect on human cells as they have on bacteria. However, nobody seems to worry about this, and as long as there is no proof beyond doubt that some of these additives are really dangerous for our health, the authorities will do nothing about them and their use will not be restricted. Every year more people suffer from incurable diseases whose causes are still unknown, and nobody will be able to prove that these have any relation to certain toxic substances which, for a great number of years, have often been accumulating in the human body.

Many people, especially those responsible for the prosperity of industrial enterprises, point out that the extremely small quantities of additives being used are completely harmless. But there is now plenty of proof, for example in the case of homoeopathic remedies, that the human organism can react strongly to infinitely small quantities of toxic or non-toxic substances. Even Catherine de Medici killed her enemies using only the smallest amounts of poison!

The human body has not been equipped with anything which could be used to detoxify the ever-growing quantity of foreign substances we ingurgitate day by day. Parts of these cannot be excreted and remain somewhere in the body, where they start to accumulate. These substances hinder metabolism as well as many other functions of the organism, and very little is known at present about what might happen when different toxins come into contact with each other, causing dangerous inter-reactions. Although in medicine we have known about these problems for many decades, the industry completely ignores the fact that such reactions could be detrimental to our health.

CHAPTER THREE

Fluids

Addictive and unsuitable drinks

Many people nowadays prefer to drink coffee, black tea, hot chocolate, soft drinks, cola drinks, alcoholic drinks and perhaps also milk, which is often quite indigestible, instead of water.

Coffee and other drinks containing caffeine stimulate the taste buds in the mouth. They also stimulate the digestive juices in the stomach, increase the heartbeat and the functions of the brain, help temporarily against migraine headache and stimulate urine production and bowel movement. These reactions may last only a few minutes or sometimes for several hours. Then the counter-reaction starts. The coffee drinker becomes more and more nervous and sometimes shaky, melancholic or depressive. Habitual coffee drinking can be the cause of serious or chronic migraines.

Sugar addiction and coffee addiction are very similar. The coffee drinker tends to drink coffee very often and some people drink up to eight cups of coffee, or even more, per day. In the long run coffee is a nerve poison; cola drinks which contain much caffeine are often the cause of the highly strung state of some children. Sleeplessness and depression are only some of the problems from which coffee drinkers suffer.

After the consumption of alcoholic drinks there are similar reactions and those who make a habit of drinking alcohol may be creating severe health problems for themselves. Since the First World War the consumption of coffee and sweet drinks has increased tenfold, and the number of alcoholics is frightening. Because coffee and alcohol stimulate kidney function and water elimination from the reserves of the body, these kinds of drinks can really dry out the body.

Most children like to drink chocolate drinks. Professor Mommsen, a well-known German paediatrician, wrote on this subject: 'Chocolate drinks often contain between 60–70 per cent of sugar and for this reason should be rejected. These drinks also contain quite indigestible cacao, caffeine and saturated fats.'

Chocolate can provoke serious allergies, and the degree of saturation is so high that when children eat or drink chocolate they often will lose their natural appetite. The biggest problem is that these drinks do not contain the natural complementary substances which enable chocolate milk to be properly digested. (The same applies to plain chocolate, which is a vitamin and mineral robber.) However, these kinds of breakfast drinks sell very well and are very popular. Business always comes before health and may even be legally protected.

Most children, when they are thirsty, prefer to ask for

sweet drinks. Although at first some of these drinks are thirst-quenching, after a short time the child again becomes thirsty, because of the sugar content in these drinks. Of course, this is the intention of the manufacturer. When thirsty one should drink water – nothing but fresh, natural water.

HOW MUCH SHOULD WE ACTUALLY DRINK?

'You ought to drink more! At least two litres per day!' Quite often we hear this well-meant advice. The general opinion that we should drink at least two litres per day stems from a very simple calculation. On average our body excretes daily about two and a half litres of liquid. Of course, one then assumes that this loss of water has to be replaced. However, we forget that some food contains much liquid. Some natural foods, like fruit, vegetables or rice, can contain more than 90 per cent of water.

What were things like in primeval times? Did people at that time also make sure to drink at least two litres daily? Certainly not! In those times they had no soft drinks or cola drinks, nor coffee or tea. Even water was not always available. But this was not as important as it seems, as those people lived exclusively on natural food which was full of water. Besides, in the tropical forests there were many plants which contained liquid. Even today there is a palm tree in the tropics which is called 'the travellers' palm tree'. Its leaves contain so much water that several people can drink sufficiently from it.

Animals such as rabbits, who eat 100 per cent raw food,

drink hardly anything. The first primitive peoples did not eat any salt, sugar or other concentrated food, with the possible exception of very small quantities of honey.

Our bodies can only process such concentrated food when it has been diluted first. For this reason we get thirsty when we eat anything which is concentrated. Our brain regulates this process automatically. As nowadays we consume more and more concentrated food, we are usually more thirsty. Modern people have to drink plenty, otherwise they would become dehydrated. We can no longer live like our ancestors.

How frequently one has to drink, and the amount of liquid one needs, is something very personal. It depends on how much we eat and what we eat, on our age and on several other factors. What is enough for one person may be insufficient for another. Somebody who eats in a way which nowadays is considered normal will need more liquid than a vegetarian who lives mainly on raw vegetables and little cooked food. The more concentrated food such as salt or sugar one eats, the more one needs to drink. Bread is also a highly concentrated food. Have you ever noticed that birds, when they eat bread, need lots of water? Athletes and people who work physically and perspire a lot need more water than people who sit at their desks all day every day. In summer, we need more liquid than we do in the winter. When the weather is dry we need more liquid than when it is humid.

As long as we are still young, we know when we are thirsty. The older we become, the less we notice when we ought to drink. Therefore, at a certain age one has to be careful not to drink too little. We need at least one and a half litres per day! However, one should not drink just anything. Most modern drinks are no thirst-quenchers. We only drink these modern drinks to please our taste buds and sometimes, as an exception to the rule, we may enjoy an occasional cup of coffee or tea. But the only healthy drink is water, nothing but water. We should not overdo this either, though. We need water, but not in too large quantities. It is said that water cleans and flushes the kidneys. That is true, but excessive liquid puts too much stress on your kidneys and can have disastrous consequences. You should always keep to the happy medium and try to estimate yourself how much water on average you need per day.

OUR BODIES NEED WATER

Our planet consists of 70 per cent water, and all life on earth depends upon this water. The human body also consists mainly of water. All body fluids, like urine, blood, lymphatic fluid, perspiration, tears, saliva, the fluids in our joints, gastric juices etc., contain water, lots of water. In our body tissues and in every body cell there is water. Water plays an important part in the transfer of information and other processes in our body.

The human embryo consists of 85 per cent water and the water content of the body of a child is still very high. Later the water content decreases and can finally be reduced to about 45 per cent at a very old age. Some elderly people really look 'dried out'. As the feeling of being thirsty diminishes the older we become, the bodies of many elderly people are continuously under-supplied with water and many diseases are linked with water loss in the body. Not only the body but also the brain suffers from a lack of water. Drinking more water and doing mental exercises like so-called 'brain-jogging' can help to slow down this process.

When we are in water we feel good, and a shower gives us new energy. Before we were born we lived for nine months in an amniotic fluid and all body cells live in a watery environment. Therefore we need good, pure water and this water in our bodies needs to be replaced and supplied continuously. During our lives we need water externally as well as internally. Where there is a lack of water, there is also a lack of energy; not only coffee, but also water gives tired people a temporary high.

DISTILLED WATER

Nowadays one hears and reads more and more about distilled water. This is water that has been intensively cleansed by steaming and does not contain any harmful substances. It can, on the contrary, absorb from the body inorganic minerals and harmful substances, so that these can be excreted. Because of this many healers and also some physicians recommend that patients drink only distilled water.

It certainly would not hurt you to drink, for example, once a year for a few weeks only distilled water. But it should not be done for too long a period, as this practice has not only positive but also negative points. Firstly, such water flushes out not only pollutants but also substances that may be important for our health. Secondly, this kind of water is not natural water, as it contains hardly any life-giving substances.

For all our bodily functions we need positive as well as negative energy waves or, as the Chinese say, yin and yang. So I do not suggest that only organic minerals are good for us and inorganic minerals are bad. Healthy water contains organic as well as inorganic minerals and in this way the balance of all ingredients, and an optimal energy supply, is guaranteed. Scientists still argue about this topic, but many things still remain unknown.

Due to our unnatural lifestyle, more and more toxic waste products accumulate in our body. So it would certainly be advisable to do something about this from time to time. A treatment with distilled water can be very beneficial for our health. Many people feel rejuvenated and have more energy after such a cure. Several thousand years before our time, people drank only natural water, which contained many substances they needed and their average health was, without any doubt, much better than ours. Although arteriosclerosis and other diseases of civilisation are mainly caused by the consumption of too much protein and refined carbohydrates, it is a known fact that most people who suffer from these diseases do not drink enough water. Water can flush many harmful substances out of the body.

The most important thing is always to drink water which is as natural and as pure as possible. Natural spring and well water, unfortunately, have become a rare luxury.

Although outside of Europe and the USA it can seldom be recommended to drink tap water, most of us tend to believe that in the United States and most European countries the quality of the drinking water is strictly controlled and completely safe. However, it is extremely difficult to prevent water pollution and although the water authorities try to do their best, it is hardly possible for them to keep the tap water clean, as contaminants are increasing all the time.

In the US and Europe there are thousands and thousands of miles of water ducts that have been in use for more than a hundred years, and it is impossible to replace these all at once. Many of these ducts leak and such leaking always goes both ways, so that innumerable toxins can get into our tap water. Water pollution can come from human and animal waste, industrial discharge, fertilisers, pesticides, chemicals, nitrates, metals, foreign bodies and, always, more and more dangerous bacteria and other organisms as well as from products from septic tanks, plumbing, brass fixtures, batteries, mining, smelting and so on. Many of these substances may find their way into our water supply and cleansing procedures cannot cope with all of them. These toxins can cause gastroenteritis infections, kidney and nervous system damage, liver damage, skin problems, birth defects, cancer, brain damage and much more. Only some of the harmful bacteria and organisms can be killed by boiling the water, and doing so does not affect most metals and chemicals.

It is advisable to buy bottled drinking water in glass bottles, as the water deteriorates quickly in plastic bottles.

After buying water in plastic bottles one should, as soon as possible, pour it into a glass container.

Salt

Our bodies need salt – but what kind of salt?

When we think of fluids we also think of salt, because salt helps the body to retain fluid.

Several years ago, after many complicated calculations, scientists found out how much salt (inorganic sodium chloride) we need daily. They measured the content of the salt in the blood and tissues, and subtracted the amount of salt which is excreted through the urine and perspiration. They then found out that we need, at the most, seven to eight grams of salt a day.

In reality, however, many people consume five or six times this amount. In Japan, where heart diseases are common, the consumption of salt is even higher – up to 50 or 60 grams per day. That is between 10 and 18 kilograms of salt per year!

Almost all food sold in the supermarket contains salt. There is not only hidden sugar, but also much hidden salt in many kinds of food. Most of us have no idea how much salt we consume every day. When eating snacks or cocktail tidbits, we often become very thirsty. Too much salt is very harmful; it should be diluted with water as soon as possible before it causes too much damage.

Unfortunately, many people, especially older people, fail to realise anymore how thirsty they really are. Salt crystals in the body cause the body tissues to swell and the blood pressure will then go up. Consuming too much salt also affects the kidneys; they are no longer able to excrete such large amounts of salt, with the result that the salt goes back into the body tissues and causes dropsy, fluid retention, kidney diseases and the clogging of the capillaries. One can observe this in the little red veins which appear on the face or the legs and ankles of elderly people.

Through eating too much salt, the 260 taste buds (receptors) in the mouth can gradually become paralysed. They do not react anymore; the person in question no longer notices the salty taste of the food. Automatically, such a person will eat more and more salt and thus becomes a salt addict. Healthy food should always be prepared with plenty of savoury and aromatic herbs. In most restaurants the tiresome preparation of herbs, except perhaps in some gourmet restaurants, has long been given up. Using salt is much easier and this, of course, has the added advantage of making the clients thirsty, so that they will order more drinks. Abuse of salt has become a habit in many private kitchens as well.

But please do not make the mistake of eating food which is completely salt-free; that is just as bad as having too much salt. Natural salt (sodium chloride), which is mainly contained in fruit and vegetables, is a valuable substance, which must not be confused with the inorganic common salt mentioned earlier. In combination with other biological substances, natural sodium chloride is the most important ingredient of the lymphatic fluid and is needed for the transference of nerve impulses in the body. Salt water conducts the finest electrical currents and therefore normal blood serum contains a high percentage of sodium chloride. For the production of saliva and gastric juices or for the metabolism of fats, this natural salt is always needed.

If you are eating too much salt and wish to eat healthier, the best thing you can do is to use herbal salts or sea salt in the future, as these are less dangerous than table salt. Common table salt has been mined from deep in the earth. The natural mineral salts it contained originally have slowly trickled out and become lost, leaving only inorganic concentrated salt, which is quite indigestible. Sea salt is an alternative but this, too, is very concentrated and although less harmful than common table salt, should be used only in small quantities.

MILK

Do we need milk?

Humans are the only creatures who drink milk alien to their species, even when they are grown up, although their organism is not equipped to digest it adequately. It is a known fact that adult milk drinkers are to be found mostly in industrialised countries, where the percentage of caries of the teeth, hip-joint operations and diseases of the bones are the highest. Most surprisingly, many people in Africa and Asia, who never drink milk, have strong teeth and healthy bones.

Only a small percentage of the world's population drinks cow's milk. In antiquity and during the Middle Ages, cheese, especially goat's cheese, was eaten at times, but drinking milk was not a common habit and goat's milk was usually only an emergency solution when feeding babies. Later, cow's milk was used only sporadically until about a hundred years ago. Then, scientists discovered that milk contained many valuable substances. Since then dairy products have grown into a billion-dollar industry and milk is recommended as one of the healthiest foods, even by many doctors.

Of course, raw, untreated cow's milk contains many vital substances. But it seems no one has realised that any food is only good for our health if our organism can metabolise it. Unfortunately, with cow's milk this is often not the case. The problem with milk is that as soon as it comes into contact with oxygen, or has been heated or treated (pasteurised etc.) in any way, its originally valuable ingredients change and become totally different substances. Many people have an allergic reaction to this milk and are unable to metabolise the milk proteins or the milk sugar. The following section explains why this is so.

THE DIFFERENCE BETWEEN MOTHER'S MILK AND COW'S MILK

Mother's milk is the ideal food for any baby. But there are many different kinds of milk and each kind has a different composition. Horse's milk contains exactly what the foal needs; goat's milk is good for the little kid etc. Every mammal on earth needs, exclusively, the milk from its own kind. A calf grows much faster than a human baby and because of this, cow's milk contains much more calcium, phosphorus and protein than human milk.

Mother's milk contains almost twice as much milk sugar as cow's milk, but the quality of the milk sugar is totally different; mother's milk contains mainly lactose. This lactose is instrumental in developing bacterial flora, which is much needed in the baby's intestines to protect the baby from illness. Also, lactose is indispensable for the body's own production of myelin, a kind of fat that surrounds the nerve fibres. When these nerves are not protected enough, serious mental (nervous) diseases, like multiple sclerosis, can develop. Scientists in New Zealand have researched these connections in great detail. Also, leukaemia and some kinds of cancer seem to link with the consumption of cow's milk.

The fat content of mother's milk and cow's milk is almost the same, but there is a great difference in quality here also. Mother's milk contains more specific fatty acids, which are very important for the development of the nerves and the brain. A baby fed only on cow's milk grows faster and often gains more weight than a baby who drinks mother's milk. However, a breast-fed baby usually has no digestive problems, its defence system functions better and its mental and spiritual development is superior.

In the stomach of a newborn baby there are completely different enzymes from those found in the stomachs of small children and grown-ups. As the baby grows, the composition of the gastric juices gradually changes. After this the digestive system is prepared to handle a different kind of food.

THE CONNECTIONS BETWEEN CLIMATIC CONDITIONS AND MILK COMPATIBILITY

In this section I would like to expand a little on the paragraphs on this subject in Chapter 1.

In southern countries, where the sun is nearly always shining and people eat more fish, an excellent calcium supply is practically guaranteed. In Asia and other countries, where people do not drink milk, the need for calcium is covered by soy products, seaweed, seafood etc. Yet in northern countries, where the sun seldom shines and where in former times fruit and vegetables were only available during the short summer months, nature provided an emergency solution for the supply of calcium. Over many generations, people in those countries developed a gene which stimulated the production of lactose, which is needed for the digestion of milk. That is why, for instance, Scandinavians can digest milk and dairy products better than other Europeans.

Several years ago at the University of Heidelberg it was confirmed that only 55 per cent of the inhabitants of Central Europe could digest cow's milk adequately. In southern countries about 90 per cent of the population is unable to digest cow's milk completely. Unfortunately, for financial reasons, milk and dairy products are strongly promoted in these countries. This can have, as we have seen in African countries, for example, disastrous consequences. As the Third World countries still believe that the best things come from our Western countries, many doctors there recommend cow's milk as the best food for babies and small children. Most of these doctors know very little about nutrition or biological connections.

It is unbelievable how many children in countries such as Spain and Italy, under the influence of massive advertising campaigns and promotions, consume cow's milk, usually mixed with chocolate, for breakfast. Many products such as chocolate, bread, cookies, crackers etc, which contain hidden milk, do serious harm to consumers in these countries. As a result of wrong nutritional habits, many children become milk and/or sugar addicts; they become easily tired, ill or nervous and nobody seems to know why.

Perhaps some of my readers will not agree with me, as they have read that in certain warm southern countries there are people such as the Masai in Africa who not only drink milk, but practically live on it. This is true, as the Masai live mainly on milk and blood and those who still maintain these old traditions are very healthy indeed. The secret lies in the fact that they usually drink their milk straight from the udders of the cow. This milk is still completely natural. The blood comes directly from the neck artery of their cattle. Probably this kind of food would suit us better than the food we eat now.

THE DIFFERENT WAYS IN WHICH MILK IS PROCESSED

With every step of treatment the milk loses more of its original value, and it is interesting to learn what one of Germany's greatest nutritional scientists had to say about this: 'Only raw milk is *completely natural*. This kind of milk will always be the most valuable for our health. All products made from raw milk, like skimmed milk, buttermilk, whey and of course butter and fresh cream, can be regarded as *second best*, although they are still very healthy and valuable. Those can even be eaten by children and adults who otherwise have allergic reactions when eating dairy products. Butter and fresh cream contain mainly milk fat, which is easier to digest than milk protein or milk sugar.'

All types of milk which have been through a fermentation process, like sour milk, yogurt, kefir, cottage cheese and quark, provided they have been produced from raw milk, belong to the third category and can still be recommended. In the fourth category we find all heated products, e.g. pasteurised milk and dairy products made from pasteurised milk. When milk is heated, the protein molecules in the milk are damaged and this results in a loss of enzymes and vitamins. Protein in the human body is also damaged at a temperature of over 42 °C. As, however, in some countries the pasteurisation of milk is prescribed by law, one has to put up with these losses in value if one still wishes to drink milk. When milk is preserved by still higher temperatures, as it is in the case of sterilised milk and all its by-products, all vital nutrients are destroyed. They belong to the fifth category.

The next is the sixth and last category of milk preservation. This category includes condensed or tinned milk, dried milk and milk powder for babies and small children. Because of the fact that manufacturers try to make their products resemble mother's milk as much as possible, these powdered milk products receive an even more intensive treatment. Thereby the loss in valuable and vital substances increases, and those few nutrients which these products still contain undergo a complete change, compared to the original product from which they were made.

A mother who uses such milk products for her baby should realise that her baby in this way receives 'the least valuable food instead of the most valuable', to quote Professor Kollath.

WHEN BABIES CANNOT DIGEST COW'S MILK.

It often happens that babies do not have enough of the enzymes which are needed for the digestion of milk proteins. If indigestible milk residues cannot be eliminated in a normal way, the body will try to find another solution. These residues will then come out through the skin and the baby will get a skin rash, the so-called milk scab, infantile eczema, other skin problems and/or diarrhoea. If the diarrhoea or skin problems are suppressed with medicaments, this can eventually lead to the development of neurodermitis, which is very difficult to cure.

The elimination of residues from the proteins of cow's milk puts a heavy stress on the baby's kidneys, which are still underdeveloped. Milk proteins contain more than 25 different substances, which in combination with sugar or flour can trigger allergic reactions. Among these are behavioural problems, hyperactivity, nervousness, irritability and chronic fatigue, which are often evident in today's society.

If these proteins irritate the urinary tract they often cause bedwetting, even with older children. In the event of such a problem, one should try to leave milk and milk products off the menu for at least a few weeks. Often many such problems then disappear within a short time.

The habit of drinking milk

As a result of intensive publicity campaigns, milk drinking has become a general habit and many parents insist that their children drink milk regularly. People who drink milk believe that it gives them lots of calcium, which is good for their teeth and their bones. They also believe that milk prevents osteoporosis later in life. It seems that only a few people know that osteoporosis hardly exists in countries where most people never drink milk.

In Europe and North America, even adults often drink milk. As long as one does not overdo this, and as long as milk drinking does not become a daily habit, this will probably not harm them. But often it becomes an addiction, and those who are addicted to milk get a kind of 'high' each time they drink it. After a while, they have the opposite reaction and become very tired. This reaction is due to leucocytosis, which means that there is an increase of white blood cells which fight against a threat to the organism. In this case the danger lies in the milk and it is a sign that the person in question has problems digesting milk or dairy products.

Milk and osteoporosis?

Osteoporosis (atrophy of the bones) is a very complicated development in which calcium, in most cases, plays only a very minor part. On the contrary, the softening of the bones, osteomalacia, is a disease whereby, for various reasons, the deposit of calcium, vitamin B and certain phosphates in the bones is impossible, or hardly possible.

Many people, including many physicians and even the Osteoporosis Society, do not seem to know the difference between these two diseases. They still believe that it is possible to prevent and treat osteoporosis mainly by drinking milk and taking calcium tablets. However, osteoporosis is caused mainly by wrong eating habits. In that case there is often a lack of many vitamins and other vital substances, such as folic acid and vitamins C, B6, D and K (for bone growth), as well as magnesium, manganese, boron, zinc and silicon, all of which are important for the maintenance of strong and healthy bones. A lack of exercise and subsequent degeneration of the muscles, partly due to the fact that many elderly people are no longer used to lifting heavy loads, also contributes significantly to the disease. A lack of certain hormones, especially progesterone, *not* oestrogen, can play an important role in the development of osteoporosis, according to the newest research.

In the case of osteomalacia, an adequate calcium supply is extremely important. However, please note that drinking milk only helps when it is biologically controlled raw milk. Pasteurising milk or treating it even more intensively always results in a big surplus of acid, and too much acid harms bone development (bone growth). In the human body, calcium is utilised to assimilate all acids and render them inoffensive. When people often drink pasteurised or otherwise treated milk, there is so much acid in their bodies that enormous amounts of the right kind of calcium are needed in order to limit the possible damage. When milk is heated it curdles and the calcium from this milk becomes, in a qualitative sense, completely useless to us.

The best sources of calcium are vegetables, fruit, nuts,

dried fruit, and also homoeopathic and other natural remedies. Cows do not drink milk in order to give milk! Cows and other animals obtain their calcium from raw vegetables, plants and other natural foods. Also, people in other parts of the world meet their calcium needs with natural foods.

CONCLUSION

Even if you think that milk does not harm you, it would be advisable to do a simple test. You should exclude milk and milk products from your diet for about five days. (Watch out for 'hidden' milk in bread, cookies, ice cream and many other foods). After this you can test all milk and dairy products one after another by taking a small amount of one dairy product in the morning on an empty stomach, every third day. Keep it in your mouth for a little while and then swallow it. If there is no reaction (e.g. a headache) within a few hours or up to two days, you will know that this particular product is all right for you. Otherwise you should stop taking it, because it does not agree with you. Everybody is different; everyone reacts in a different way. You are, of course, free to decide whether you and your children will use milk and dairy products in the future.

Never be fanatical about your nutrition, but let common sense prevail.

CHAPTER FOUR

Blood Circulation

Many of my readers will be familiar with my lectures on the 'Five Pillars of Health'. These are nutrition, digestion, elimination, circulation and relaxation. In these lectures I often say that we must consider health as the roof of a house; this roof rests upon the five pillars, mentally, physically and emotionally. One can expect good health only if the pillars are firm.

It is a fact that when food or nutrition leads to good digestion, good absorption takes place. And that when the absorption and digestion is not right, the circulation will be affected. Nowadays I see too many problems resulting from excessive amounts of waste materials in the blood, resulting in severe problems with the blood and lymphatic systems. This in turn affects the liver, the heart, the organs and finally the cells.

Until the 19th century we knew very little about biological functions. Our knowledge is now greatly extended and we are aware that life consists of the constant renewal of cells or cellular tissue. This depends greatly upon the presence of amino acids, glucose, enzymes, vitamins, minerals and oxygen, so that the formation of cells can take place when the pillars of our house of health are strong and firm. If they are sturdy and secure, waste materials are eliminated efficiently from the body, resulting in a correctly functioning organism.

Our blood circulation depends greatly on lymphatic congestion. Every day I carry out blood tests which reveal that many patients are carrying waste materials in their blood, and this can result in many differing health problems. We must remember that the lymphatic system is very dependent upon our sleep – it is when we are sleeping that the lymphatic system carries out much of its work. Unfortunately, many people suffer from insomnia, when they not only become stressed and nervous but also succumb to illness due to the work of the lymphatic system being impaired. Some thought and close attention to the blood circulation and lymphatic system may be very helpful in maintaining and gaining better health.

HEALTHY BLOOD

Before nutrients from a healthy, well-balanced diet are absorbed into the blood, they pass through innumerable small filters, which are located in the intestinal wall. Thus the nutrients are cleaned and absorbed by the capillaries (the tiniest blood vessels). These countless capillaries, situated directly behind the intestinal wall, then come together in a wide channel, the portal vein (vena porta), which leads to the liver. The liver is our most important detoxifying organ. There the blood is again cleaned by innumerable tiny filters. It is then absorbed into the main bloodstream, together with the oxygen-containing blood which comes from the lungs.

We have two different kinds of blood, so to speak: the arterial and the venous blood. The arterial blood, which flows *from* the heart, contains all the nutrients and oxygen needed by our body cells. Its flow is almost as light as water and it has a nice red colour, due to its oxygen content. The venous blood, which flows *to* the heart, provides, along with the lymphatic fluid, the detoxification and disposal of harmful or useless materials.

The blood flows through our body in channels which become smaller and smaller. From these capillaries it finally flows into the tissues where it comes into contact with the cells. Here the so-called metabolic 'exchange' takes place. This means that the cells will now choose and absorb from the arterial blood the nutrients they need for their individual needs. On the other hand the venous blood absorbs the waste products of the cells. Certain specific waste materials are transported directly via the lymph tract to the lymphatic glands, where these materials are detoxified. Then all the different residues are transferred to the excretory organs, where they are disposed of. If, once in a while, we eat too much or indulge ourselves by eating unhealthy food, this miracle machine can repair the damage and restore health. Nobody has to be a health fanatic. Our body is a living miracle machine.

In view of the now antiquated opinion that disease is due solely to the disturbance of normal cell function (Virchow), it is known that normal cell metabolism and function depend mainly on the quality of the nutrients which are supplied by the blood.

UNHEALTHY BLOOD

Seen from a naturopath's point of view, unhealthy blood is blood of inferior quality. The quality of the blood changes when there are fluctuations in the minerals, trace elements and vitamin metabolism, when the blood fats are too high or too low, or when the protein values and the acid-alkaline metabolism and blood-clotting processes are abnormal. In that case there is always the possibility of congestion and infection.

As a result of the poor quality of most modern food, which can cause obstructions to, or permeability of, the tiny blood filters, many people today have blood of an inferior quality. These filters are able to filter only a certain amount of blood at one time, and when there are too many noxious substances, a build-up of such substances in the portal vein may develop. An accumulation of harmful substances can in turn create an accumulation of blood in the abdomen and thus be the cause of the development of a so-called 'collateral circulation'. This means that the organism, in order to prevent greater dangers, creates new blood vessels which can divert the superfluous blood. As a consequence of this haemorrhoids or varicose veins can develop, as well as the unsightly small veins on the thighs which are always an indication of blood accumulation in the larger blood vessels.

Sometimes insufficiently filtered blood can get directly into the general blood circulation. Such blood contains many irritating substances and the red blood cells in the finest blood vessels mass together, the blood cells become less mobile and blood circulation is diminished. When circulation is diminished many cells cannot be fed properly. At first the cells mainly in the periphery of the body do not get enough nutrients and the blood circulation in the feet, and often in the hands, stagnates. More and more people complain about cold feet. By and by more toxic substances are deposited in the tissues. These penetrate deep into the body and all the time more damage is done.

Bad blood circulation can also be caused by the intake of too much protein, which Professor Wendt described so well in his books and which causes very high blood pressure. It is bad for the health when one eats too much protein, mainly of animal origin; the human body is not able to use all of it. In such a case the superfluous protein is deposited in the walls of the capillaries in such a way that by and by they become clogged up and the blood can no longer pass through them. Then circulation problems, high blood pressure, hardening of the arteries, early diabetes, rheumatic diseases and gout occur. The correct therapy for these diseases would be protein fasting. In any case, the nutrition of the patient should contain very little protein and bloodletting, cupping and other natural healing methods and remedies should be prescribed (to be described in the third volume of this series).

THE IMMUNE SYSTEM

The immune system is the defence system of our body. Part of this is the lymphatic system, which is a net of lymphatic vessels similar to the layout of the blood vessels in our organism. From every part of our body toxic substances are transported via these lymph vessels to the smaller and larger lymph nodes, which are the 'sewage plants' of the organism. Bacteria, toxins, alien substances and waste products from the body itself, like dead cells and bacteria, are transported to these detoxification centres.

Some substances, e.g. those from cow's milk and certain fats, are sent directly from the intestines via the small lymph vessels, situated in the intestinal wall, to the main centre of the lymphatic defence system, situated in the abdomen. There, and in the other lymph nodes such as the tonsils and the appendix, the substances mentioned above are cleaned and detoxified. After this, all waste materials which cannot be used are taken up by the venous blood and eliminated. The most important organs through which this elimination of toxins takes place are the skin, the kidneys, the lungs and the intestines. As the greatest dangers that threaten our health develop in the abdomen, most lymphatic vessels and lymph nodes are found there. Here also a very important substance for our defence, the immune-globulin, is produced. Every second, no matter how slight the danger, millions of defensive cells are used and have to be replaced over and over again. The spleen and the thyroid gland are an important part of this defence system.

Hundreds of years ago, physicians already knew that there are many interactions between the outer skin and the inner mucus membrane which could be made use of therapeutically. There are people who have a so-called 'lymphatic constitution'. These people very often become ill when their lymphatic defences have been weakened.

They then suffer from health problems such as the common cold or a sore throat, which are nothing but a simple defence reaction of the body. Such natural reactions always have a purpose and serve to eliminate toxins.

When the health of the organism is at risk, the immune system will automatically react. One can understand this best by observing the simple defensive reactions that happen every day: if dust gets into the nose, we sneeze in order to get rid of it and protect our respiratory tract. Coughing, clearing the throat and sneezing sometimes have a double purpose: they help not only to dispose of dust particles but also to eliminate the accumulated mucus. If something gets into the eyes, tears will clean them. If we have eaten some food that does not agree with us, we get diarrhoea or we have to vomit. The main purpose of this is always the cleaning of the organism. Simple health problems will be cured by simple measures. The organism will fight greater health problems by using various and stronger defensive measures.

A lymphatic constitution is sometimes hereditary, but it is also possible to acquire such a constitution during the course of life. This can start when one is still young, for example when small children eat too many sweets or drink cow's milk. In this case the tonsils or the lymph nodes in the neck start to swell as the organism tries to neutralise the toxins. If it is not possible to neutralise all the toxins, the child may get tonsillitis (inflammation of the tonsils). It will depend upon the physician and the parents if this inflammation is treated in the correct way, by natural means, or if the child will suffer all its life from lymphatic diseases. An operation of the tonsils or a treatment with antibiotics may have serious consequences, as the tonsils can no longer act as a defensive organism. After some time other parts of the lymphatic system, such as the bronchial tubes or the mucus membranes of the sinuses, will take over those defensive functions which formerly were the task of the tonsils. If this happens and the person in question still eats an unhealthy diet, these secondary defensive systems will also become overstrained. Then, life-long chronic diseases of the bronchial system and the sinuses, as well as serious diseases of the abdomen, may develop.

Our immune system nowadays has to work non-stop at full power and is constantly overstressed. Cells of the immune system die by the million and cannot be replaced quickly enough. Innumerable alien substances, which have no place in the human body, prevent normal body functions. Any substance entering our digestive tract which cannot be used in some way means needless work for the immune system and a waste of energy.

We live in a world full of harmful substances, toxins, microbes and other tiny creatures, and each day many of these penetrate into our body. Most of the time such alien elements are rendered harmless by our defensive mechanism and are then eliminated as soon as possible. But until these facts are taught at universities, and as long as all symptoms are being suppressed regardless of causalities, there will be more and more chronic illness in the world.

Acids and Alkali

Few people, including physicians, know how harmful

acids are to our health. I have already discussed the harm acidity can do to our digestive tract and what the consequences are. Now I will repeat some of what I said, as it is extremely important for you to understand the danger. Knowing this, I am sure that you will at least give it a try to stay away from sugar and sweets and eat more vegetables and fruit, especially those that contain little acidity. You alone are responsible for your own health.

It is extremely important to know something about the most important causes of illness, and today the extreme acidity of most of our daily food stands almost at the top of the danger list. Our body needs acids, as well as alkaline mineral salts. Depending on the individual's state of health, blood has a pH value of 7.35–7.45, which should always remain more or less the same as otherwise we may become seriously ill. Each variation of this pH value will immediately be counter-balanced by the organism, in order to prevent a blockage of the veins, which can result in blood clotting, thrombosis or worse.

The urine of a healthy baby is usually very alkaline and can have a pH value of about 8. Such an alkaline value means health. As the baby grows its pH value will become more acid every year and if this value drops under 5, this baby is a very sick one. Sometimes the pH value of the urine of a person who is ill may be as low as 4, which means that his or her urine is extremely acid. Illness often occurs when there is too much acidity.

Usually, early in the morning the pH value of the first urine fluctuates between 5 or 5.5 and 7, and this you can measure yourself with small strips of prepared test paper. After dipping these strips in your urine for a few seconds you can read the result. However you will need some additional knowledge in order to be able to judge these values correctly. For example, if you have done some strenuous sports on the day before, the next morning the value of the urine might be quite acidic. While using your muscles much lactic acid can develop and this acid leaves the body early the next day. In this case the test paper may show an acid content of about 5. On the other hand, you may be a lady who just finished her monthly period, whereby much acid and many toxins have been eliminated. The organism will be in a good shape and the test strip will show a value of about 7 or over.

Animal protein produces acids but most of our daily food is overloaded with acids. At breakfast we start with rolls and jam, coffee with sugar, or white bread with sausages and ham. For lunch we eat meat with noodles or potatoes which are acidic because they have been peeled, vegetables which, because of overcooking, have a surplus of acids, salad dressings with vinegar and soft drinks. We are inundated with acids. Food which was originally alkaline becomes acid when, through industrial manipulation, it is deprived of its vital nutrients. Due to its exposure to sunlight during the ripening process most fruit is basically alkaline. However, if harvested when still unripe such fruit stays very acidic and therefore it is bad for our health. This also occurs when fruit is cooked. A natural surplus of alkali in vegetables changes into a harmful surplus of acids when these are not cooked correctly. When the cooking water is thrown away, 40–60 per cent of all minerals and 95 per cent of vitamins are lost.

Bread and cereals contain much acid. Unheated raw milk is alkaline, but as soon as it is in any way manipulated or boiled it becomes acidic. Unfortunately, with our modern food we assimilate more and more acids. The more acid there is in the body, the more serious is the disease. Too much acid can cause chronic stomach inflammation or inflammation of the intestines, and this can be the cause of flatulence, constipation and dangerous ulcers. It is also one of the main causes of rheumatic diseases.

The body tries to neutralise these acids by dissolving and withdrawing calcium and alkaline mineral salts from the bones and the teeth. As you already know, the same thing happens if these minerals are needed for the 'digestion' of white sugar, white flour and other refined foods. This leads to decalcification, and the bones lose their density and become brittle. In combination with other negative factors this can be the cause of slipped discs, tooth decay and various diseases of the bones and joints.

If you suffer from any of these problems, it is a sign that not only your urine but your entire organism is too acidic and you should try to eat as much alkaline food as possible. Many of my patients followed the advice I gave them in this respect and often the results were amazing. If your problems are not yet too serious and if you have enough staying power, you can cure yourself. In the third volume of this series you will find all the practical advice you need.

Alkaline foods are, for example, raw vegetables, bulbs, tubers, carrots, leafy vegetables, sun-ripened fruits, potatoes steamed in their skins (jacket potatoes), cold-pressed natural oil, seeds, nuts and fresh or dried herbs. Cherries are highly recommended for people suffering from rheumatic diseases. Bitter herbal teas are wonderful remedies. Most herb teas are alkaline.

By regular physical exercise, much acid can be

eliminated. Elderly people especially, who suffer most from these health problems, take little or no exercise. Taking a walk now and then does not solve the problem. Elderly people should again get into the habit of carrying small loads, so that the bones will be sufficiently burdened and strengthened. Working in the garden is very healthy. At any age muscles should be exercised regularly and it is excellent to perspire properly and abundantly at least once a day.

However, I must warn you never to overdo it. Younger people especially often tend to overdo sports. Sport is good for you and should be fun, but if people overdo it too much lactic acid is produced by the muscular exertion. This lactic acid has to be broken down and excreted from the body. If this is not possible because of a lack of minerals, the general health of the person in question will decline and they will lose their stamina. Because of this, most sporting professionals have to give up their occupation when they are still quite young. The organisms of a great number of our athletes and football stars has been inundated with acids and their stamina diminishes year by year. However, if these champions knew the origin of their problems, they could do something about it and go on for many more years.

For the same reason more and more young men become bald or semi-bald. Because of a certain lifestyle and poor eating habits, the acid content of the body increases and in order to neutralise these acids the organism takes the needed minerals from the teeth, the bones and the scalp. Hereditary disposition does not cause this unwanted baldness, the cause lies mainly with the bad eating habits of the family, which will have been the same for many generations. The other day I was reading an article in one of the best Swiss papers, the *NZZ*. The article was headed 'The consequences of evolution' and the author lamented the fact that important 'head-hunters' had stated that most men who had lost their hair had less chance to be considered for a top job than men who still had much hair. This had nothing to do with their knowledge, experience, age or other factors. According to the author of this article, becoming bald was one of the consequences of evolution. He did not know anything about the most important causes of baldness.

When we look at family pictures we see that our forebears usually had a beautiful head of hair. In those days most people did not have a lack of minerals. Many people had outdoor occupations and men did not overtire themselves playing football or other sports in order to earn millions. Baldness is one of the consequences of modern agriculture and food science, whereby most of the elements we need for our health have been scientifically removed from our soil and our daily food. Our modern way of life, too, which means sitting in an office all day long and getting too little sleep or overdoing weekend sports, has something to do with the loss of hair. Of course, hormones are also the scapegoats here, but when people are healthy and live a normal life their hormones will also behave normally.

STARCHES

There are many different harmful and useless substances which the body tries to eliminate in a natural way.

Sometimes this is not easy, especially if these substances are very sticky or very hard.

Starches are sticky and slimy and are usually found in carbohydrates such as cereals, bread and pasta, as well as in milk and dairy products, or badly processed lipids (frying fats). Normally these starches are eliminated via the liver, the intestines or the sebaceous glands of the skin. However, when there are too many starches the excretory organs are overburdened, and other ways will be found to dispose of them. For example, the respiratory tract or the mucus lining of the uterus are suitable for such disposals and the starches will then leave the organism in the form of mucus or as a white discharge. When the organism becomes saturated with too many starches you may get a running nose, a cold and a sore throat. Diseases such as asthma, bronchitis, wet eczema, acne, inflammation of the uterus (endometriosis) and the digestive organs can develop. In this case the mucus is mostly thick and viscous.

THE TREATMENT

A change of diet or even fasting, or a so-called 'dry diet', can always be recommended. Often the mistake is made to advise such patients 'to drink as much as possible'. However, this kind of advice is completely wrong, as much liquid is only needed in the case of feverish diseases; liquids thin the blood and the fever goes down. But in the case of the above-mentioned health problems or diseases, the accumulation of mucus is the greatest problem and starches are not soluble in water.

All diseases whereby starches and mucus play an

important part point to a weakness of the lymphatic system and the lymphatic nodes may become inflamed. If there are too many starches in the food, the defensive forces can hardly cope with all the work. In order to prevent or cure such a disease, it is very important to stop eating starches and to put an end to the build-up of the mucus-producing waste products mentioned above.

The quantity of blood should always be more or less the same. When a patient suffers from one of the above-mentioned diseases, it would be wise to keep the intake of liquids to a minimum. Then the organism will compensate for this deficiency by using the liquid contained in the lymphatic nodules. In order to achieve this, the lymphatic nodules will be squeezed out and emptied and after a short time the liquid in these nodules will be replaced by newly made lymphatic fluids. This kind of therapy means a real house-cleaning, as in this way superfluous mucus can be eliminated, the lymphatic nodes will be cleaned and the disease can be cured. This is a 'dry diet', which is a diet whereby for a few days the patient takes only a minimum of fluids. Such a treatment is usually quite successful.

CRYSTALS

Diseases caused by too much mucus usually do not hurt. On the other hand, diseases which result from crystallisation can be extremely painful. We know that crystallisation takes place when certain solutions become saturated. Crystals are as hard as a needle and in the human body they consist mainly of urea and uric acids, which come essentially from animal protein like meat, fish, eggs, milk and milk products. They can come also from acidic fruits, cereals and leguminous plants.

Normally crystals can be eliminated by way of the kidneys and the sweat glands of the skin. However, you should know that, for example, the kidneys are able only to excrete a certain amount of uric acid in 24 hours. Nowadays, our nutrition contains too much protein and acidic food and drinks, and the normal systems of elimination are overstrained. Our body consists of about 70 per cent liquid and as soon as there are too many different kinds of acid, especially uric acid, in our body, crystallisation begins. After some time many crystals are then deposited in the skin, the joints, the kidneys, the gall bladder etc. Subsequently dry eczema, back problems, lumbago, sciatica, gallstones, kidney stones, kidney diseases and inflammations can develop. Acidity and the formation of crystals are the main causes not only of all kinds of rheumatic diseases but also of inflammations, ulcers, heart disease and blood circulation problems and literally hundreds of other health problems.

Every time our organism is saturated with different acids, condensation takes place and, for example, uric acid which was formerly in a liquified state changes into the hard crystals of uric acid salts. As soon as this crystallisation takes place, the pain begins. This pain is due to crystals which press on sensitive nerves. When the weather is cold the blood flows slower, especially in certain parts of the body like the hands and the feet, and often the deposits of crystals and rheumatic pain start here.

The treatment

Because of fermentation of the food mush in the intestinal tract, the intestines often contain much acid. It is therefore extremely important to prevent such fermentation.

The best way to prevent a major breakdown of your health is a protein fast and all food that contains no, or very little, protein is recommended. Furthermore, you should stay away from any food producing acidity, especially sugar and citrus fruits, anything prepared with vinegar and all the unnatural food I mentioned before. There are many different natural treatments, as well as herbs, which will help to dilute and eliminate crystals.

If you want to know if you are eating the right food, it would be advisable to check your morning urine once in a while. By using the little test papers which are sold for this purpose, you can find out if your urine is too acidic. If this is the case, you should change your eating habits and take once or twice a day some basic powder which your pharmacist will recommend, or Centauriun.

CHAPTER FIVE

RELAXATION

I have written many books on the subject of relaxation. One can relax through swimming, cycling, walking, yoga, aerobics, golfing, the Alexander Technique, and there are many more techniques and therapies that we could list. It is not my intention to write about various forms of relaxation here. My main aim is that we know, with our busy daily schedules, that we should relax more often. We need to sit down and perhaps meditate or ensure that the body at least gets a chance to recover from our daily stresses.

Sleep is very important and I will discuss this in the next chapter. In addition, the body requires a further form of relaxation. Often a workaholic will say that his work *is* his relaxation, because it is his hobby. Nevertheless, he or she forgets that there is a slow and gradual build-up of tension within the body and many illnesses are the result of stress when the body does not receive the opportunity to relax. I have seen many cancer patients who have become the victims of stressful situations. A cancerous cell is very much like a brain cell – it requires rest and meditation. When I look at my old friends who are well over 100 years of age, I am amazed at how relaxed and balanced they are in their approach to life. This reinforces my belief that it is of the utmost importance to find the correct balance, knowing when to stop and give the body a rest.

Stress and disease are common at the beginning of this new millennium. I often recall that, according to Dr Hans Seleye, we all need a measure of stress. Normal stress is a challenge, which strengthens the body's own defences. However, abnormal stress and too much stress, from which millions of people in the industrial countries suffer, can overtax us physically as well as mentally.

THE NATURAL BALANCE IS BEING DESTROYED

Health and illness are based on very specific natural laws, which must always be observed. These laws concern the constant changes of being awake and sleeping, day and night, work and relaxation, happiness and sadness and so on.

Formerly, people were obliged to go early to bed and get up early. In those times daily life depended on daylight and candles were expensive. In our time, there are many people who do not go to sleep before midnight and even later. As our organism still reacts to natural sources of light, this habit usually has a negative effect on our nervous system.

Money and Possessions

In our industrial countries there are millions of people who work only in order to earn the money they need for their livelihood. They do not care for the work as such and this can be considered a very negative stress factor. Unfortunately, although most people now earn much more than ever before, this does not improve their health.

Apart from normal daily expenses, what do people do with their money? They often buy things they like, but do not really need. By making things their possession, they try to build up their 'image'. This means they want to impress friends and neighbours that they are doing well, according to the principle that 'people who have many possessions are very clever and should be admired'. The more primitive a person is, the more he wants to possess and to buy. Therefore he always needs more money and has to work harder. In this way, uncountable people get into an unheeded and constant stress situation.

Work and Relaxation

People who work should also relax. However, many people think that relaxation equates with modern entertainment like television, visiting nightclubs, or holidays which often are far too strenuous and bring no relaxation. People eat and drink too much and many of them try to forget their problems through intoxicating amusement. When caught up in the vicious circle of modern entertainment, this brings more disadvantages than advantages. One has only to think about bad television programmes or about the so-called 'modern sports' which deal more with sensation and business than with real sport. In order not to lose the taste for it, the different stimuli have to be increased all the time. The stimuli of today become the boredom of tomorrow and we hardly know any satisfaction. Real relaxation does not seem to exist any more. Delight because of beautiful things and the adventure of living are known only to a few.

Although young people still spent part of their time in the fresh air, often the oxygen inhaled during the day will be wasted in the nightclubs and sometimes hearing will be harmed irreparably. In the same way the businessman tries to compensate for unhealthy living habits such as sedentary lifestyle and many business dinners. He goes jogging or does some other weekend sport, which will hardly make him healthy. Many people suffer more and more from unhealthy stress situations.

REFUGEES AND IMMIGRANTS

Many refugees and immigrants from, for example, Eastern Europe and the Third World become ill because of fear, stress and homesickness. There is another reason for their susceptibility to illness: the unusual food. When observing our fellow human beings at the supermarket, we may see that these newcomers often load up their shopping carts with many foods which we seldom buy. As soon as these people earn more money than they were used to, most of their earnings will be used to buy food.

This stems partly from an unconscious fear of going hungry and also from the fact that many people still think that to eat great quantities of food improves health. It is a fact that carbohydrates often give a sense of security, safety and consolation. As for these people quantity is very important and they do not know anything about the quality of the unfamiliar products they buy – everything looks so nice – many of them not only become mentally but also physically ill. The stress of foreign food has been added to their mental stress. Who will help these people?

FRIGHT

People are often frightened, and often their fears are totally unfounded. Everybody should examine their fears and try to imagine what would happen if what they fear really happened. Dale Carnegie wrote that things hardly ever become as bad as we fear. In most cases fright brings about unheeded stress, which only harms us.

Excess stress can result in a build-up of toxicity, which can lead to many problems. We only need to look at irritable bowel syndrome, which is basically the result of a combination of an incorrect diet and stress. These factors result in a toxic condition being formed in the bowel. The bowel reacts against this and if we do not address the warning, further problems can occur. Why not look towards one's diet or take a good antioxidant? Alternatively, taking several different remedies can quickly resolve the situation. In addition, do not forget that there are many non-addictive preparations that can be taken to eliminate the extra stress or nervous anxiety, or ease the unconscious turmoils inviting and causing the onset of health problems and disease.

CHAPTER SIX

SLEEP

Sleep is one of the most wonderful things. I am often asked how I manage to work 90 hours a week. My answer is quick – I have a God-given ability to sleep whenever and wherever I wish. If my body is exhausted, I can go off and have a sleep. After just half an hour of sleep, I feel fully energised.

The biggest concern I have today is for those who cannot sleep. Certainly one person will require less or more sleep than the next, but I still advocate that the majority of people should have seven to eight hours' sleep a night. I greatly admired my old partner, Dr Alfred Vogel, as he was usually in bed by nine o'clock, or at the latest ten o'clock. He worked on the principle that the hours before midnight were more valuable to the body than the hours after. He would then arise at four or five o'clock in the morning to work in the garden or to answer the hundreds of letters he received.

As we have been reading, the lymphatic system does a superb job in cleansing our blood. If there is too much waste material in our lymph glands we can experience problems. Very often, the tired people who come along to my clinics are suffering from this. Lymph swellings are full of toxic materials, resulting in the system being unable to function properly. This is often the case with ME patients, especially those that have suffered glandular fever.

During one's sleep, the lymphatic system should be cleansed. If one cannot sleep, it is wise to take a natural remedy such as Doctor Vogel's Valerian-Hops, at a dose of 30 drops, half an hour before going to bed. Alternatively, it would be beneficial to take a very good antioxidant preparation, such as Daily Choice Antioxodant or Michael's Antidoxidant, to help clear the lymphatic system. It is imperative that you ensure your lymphatic system is functioning to its maximum ability. If it isn't, you should consult a qualified and experienced doctor or practitioner for guidance. I have seen numerous illnesses and disease develop from a congested lymphatic system.

In general, many people have forgotten how to live. The worst thing for a non-sleeper is to stay up late watching an exciting television programme. This results in the mind being over-stimulated and over-excited. Cheese and crackers is often the late-night supper that accompanies a late television programme; unfortunately, this will only exacerbate the situation as cheese eaten late adversely influences the sleep pattern. Instead of eating a large supper, with meat products being the biggest culprit, insomniacs should drink a cup of herbal tea such as Melissa or Dutch herbal tea.

One interesting factor I have observed in vegetarians is that they are usually good sleepers. Up to now I have not said a lot about meat, but I would like to discuss it now, as

I feel that its effect on our nervous system results in a detrimental effect on our sleeping pattern.

In the past, meat was quite different from what it is now. Then, a healthy animal which grazed on unpolluted grass or was hunted provided much healthier meat than that which is available today. For a long time meat was a luxury which most people could not afford. Later it gradually became cheaper and now almost everyone can afford it. Today meat has been given the place of honour; vegetables and other foods do not seem to be quite so important anymore for most people who live in the industrial countries.

Do we need meat or does it interfere with our sleep?

There are millions of people in the world who do not eat meat and are nevertheless healthy. Eating is something very personal, and eating meat is no exception. Although the meat we eat today is certainly not one of our healthiest foods, there are people who obviously need the satisfaction which they derive from eating it. It seems to give them a pleasure one could call addictive. If these people do not eat meat more than twice a week, it probably will not harm them; the pleasure they find in eating will counterbalance the possible negative effects meat may have on their health. Here 'mind over matter' is very important.

Many religions do not permit the consumption of pork. This is not only for religious reasons but also for reasons of health. Pork contains much fat and provides ideal living conditions for germs and viruses; it can therefore cause all kinds of diseases. For this reason pork, and all products made from pork, is definitely not a healthy food.

EATING MEAT CAN CAUSE ILLNESS

Since meat has become cheaper, its consumption has increased phenomenally. There are people who eat up to 80 kilograms or even more meat per year. The human organism does not have the ability to process such vast amounts of meat.

As soon as an animal has been killed its meat starts to decompose and, because of this, the bodies of meat-eaters constantly dispatch leucocytoses, part of the body's defensive system to fight the invading bacteria. Their stools usually smell foul. Many meat-eaters suffer often from constipation, as muscle meat lacks fibre.

With the aid of a capillary microscope one can see that the capillaries are often damaged as a consequence of eating meat. During an average lifetime, the net of these tiny blood vessels shrinks from initially 100,000 kilometres to about 50,000.

When meat is digested much acid develops, and this puts a great deal of strain on the liver and the kidneys. These acids are stored as crystals in the body tissues and later they enter the cells and cause gout, rheumatism, diabetes, obesity, kidney diseases and neuralgia (see 'Crystals' in Chapter 5).

Which meat does most harm?

It has been known for a long time that pork and everything which is made from it, such as bacon, ham, sausages etc., is bad for our health and the latest scientific research reveals that poultry and veal are also not good for us. These meats seem to dissolve very quickly in the human body and can, within a short time, inundate the blood with so much acid that even the healthiest body cannot cope with it.

The quality of meat can vary greatly. The meat of an animal which has roamed about the Argentine pampas and eaten food which is 100 per cent natural is certainly much healthier than that of an animal raised in an industrial country which receives, twice a day, its portion of so-called 'power-fodder'. In the past such special food consisted of cereals and other natural products like soybeans, which fulfilled the needs of the animals in an optimal way. However, recently, until only a few years ago, the major part of a this 'power-fodder' not only endangered the health of the animals but also could cause very serious diseases in millions of human beings.

Concentrated fodder and disease

Could you imagine a lion living on grass and vegetables? Certainly not! Very soon such a lion would become seriously ill and die. Everybody is able to understand this. Lions are carnivores, meat-eaters, and their digestive organs cannot digest other food. On the other hand, grass and raw vegetables are completely right for cows and other herbivorous animals. Cows are plant-eaters and their digestive system, with its three stomachs, has been exclusively made to digest grass and other greens. If a cow swallows a few ants or beetles it will not come to any harm.

However, a few decades ago profit-conscious manufacturers came up with an idea which is not only extremely dangerous but also quite unbelievable. In order to make more money, they began to treat cows and other plant-eaters like carnivorous animals! Cows can now eat meat! Many people cannot believe this, but it is the truth. Of their own accord cows would never even touch meat, so some years ago manufacturers came up with the wonderful idea of a trick, a deception, so that cows would not know what they were eating. (By the way, the same trick has been used for a long time to fool people, in the use of artificial additives, especially phospates.) Foul-tasting and smelling meat residues and remains are, by using flavourings that are exactly adapted to the taste of the animals, changed into *real* gourmet food for cows and the cows love it! This special power-fodder guarantees, because of its very high protein content, that calves will grow very fast, cattle will gain much weight, and cows will give far more milk – up to 15 litres per day!

This kind of fodder has become big business, and at the same time industry has been able to solve two serious problems:

1. As meat consumption has, during the last 100 years, increased at least five times, the disposal of millions of animal carcasses, which in the past was very costly and troublesome, is now very profitable.
2. Concentrated food made from soy or cereals is very expensive and most of it has to be imported. Therefore

animal waste processing became a booming business.

Everywhere in the Western world there are recycling plants where dead animals and meat residues are made into meal for animal fodder. These are horrible places, very dirty and evil-smelling, where fat, blood, intestines, bones, heads and tails, as well as the entire bodies, of cows, pigs, sheep, chickens and other animals are processed. Although the dead animals are checked at random to ascertain if they were healthy, it is quite impossible to detect certain diseases in the initial stage and there always remains a certain risk of infectious diseases.

THE WRONG FUEL

No animal can stay healthy when it is forced to eat food it cannot really digest. The same thing happens as when the engine of a car is given the wrong type of fuel. Gradually the engine will deteriorate and eventually break down. A young calf which is fed with the above-mentioned power-fodder will grow faster, but it will never be as healthy as a calf which gets the right fodder. Such an animal loses its natural defences against all kinds of bacteria and infections. On the one hand, these animals get too much protein; on the other hand, this alien food lacks many of the essential nutrients cows need in order to be healthy.

Although cows now give more milk and cattle put on more muscle, they are no longer strong and healthy animals. They are ill more often and need more and more antibiotics and other drugs. Some of these are prohibited and can only be obtained on the black market. Many of these medicaments cannot be completely broken down in the body of the animal, and when we eat meat or drink milk a small part of these will be assimilated in our body.

THE DANGER INCREASES – BSE

In the beginning, people were not worried about possible infections from the meat of animals fed on power-fodder. Animal farming was doing well and the animals seemed to be quite healthy. Then, about 25 years ago, more and more cattle started to suffer from BSE, also known as 'mad cow disease' (bovine spongiform encephalopathy). It then came to light that sheep which were infected with this illness had eaten contaminated power-fodder. Cattle and other animals, even those in zoos and domestic cats, which had also eaten contaminated fodder, became ill and died. More and more veterinarians and scientists became very concerned about what was happening.

Animals suffering from this illness showed the typical symptoms of a cerebral disease. They became nervous and vicious; their whole bodies trembled. No longer were they able to co-ordinate their movements. After a while they collapsed and died. Soon BSE became a catastrophe which was more and more widespread. In England a well-known nutrition expert demanded the slaughter of millions of cattle. Actually only about a quarter of a million were killed, which even then almost brought about a crisis in the British government. The first BSE cases were reported in some European countries which had been importing English cattle for many years.

BSE is an encephalopathy, a disease of the brain, which can be transferred orally, that is via food. The BSE epidemic, especially in Great Britain, had been spreading more and more and after some years, in 1990, it was realised that there was also an unusual increase of a certain cerebral disease in people. This disease is called Creuzfeld-Jacob Disease, CJD for short, and it affects the central nervous system. Although it was officially denied that BSE and CJD had anything to do with each other, it was very frightening all the same. We know that CJD can take 20 years to develop and although many known scientists seemed to be sure that it is impossible for humans to be infected with BSE, other experts were not convinced of this. Scientific research revealed that many animals suffering from BSE showed the same symptoms as those found in people who have certain diseases of the brain, not only in the case of CJD, but also when people have Alzheimer's disease or multiple sclerosis – in all these diseases some parts of the brain show an extensive degeneration of brain cells.

Such diseases are probably not infectious diseases in the usual sense, as there are no normal reactions of the immune system in order to fight the infection. As far as is currently known, hereditary disposition has little to do with this and many scientists therefore agree that these diseases are caused by up-to-now unknown disease-provoking mechanisms. It is absolutely logical that all animals, including cattle, cannot be healthy and will, after some time, become chronically ill when eating the wrong kinds of food, which they cannot digest. The meat of weak and diseased animals can never be healthy for us, and when these animals have somehow become infected by the meat of other diseased animals, it is far worse.

The big problem is that the incubation period, that is the

time it takes from the earliest beginning until the actual development of a disease, can be very long. It can take several years for a diseased animal to be diagnosed, although this animal may already have been ill for some time. It is almost impossible to prevent the transmission of such diseases.

Some years ago, after quite sensational media coverage of this problem, people became very frightened and many no longer wished to eat meat at all. But after a while things got back to normal and it seemed that the danger had passed. Was there really no more danger? Nobody knew for sure. The authorities certainly took adequate measures to protect the public, but still nobody knew exactly what fodder cattle and other slaughter animals were being fed in their home countries or abroad. Did they now get the expensive soy or cereal fodder? How many animal waste-processing plants (knacker's yards) were originally in Europe and North America? Were some of these still operating? Which imported meat, from which countries, came or still comes from healthy animals?

Did cows finally get used to the idea of being treated like carnivorous animals? Of course, they will never get used to it and in consequence all the animals which are fed in this way will degenerate and, in the long run, become diseased. Although the danger of BSE seems to have passed, at least for the moment, there is a still greater danger – the ignorance and stupidity of people who think they know better than nature.

Many questions are still open. Questions which apparently are not important anymore. Meanwhile the increase of brain and nervous diseases has become frightening. Could there be a connection between those diseases and certain eating habits? Why was hardly any scientific research done in this area? You can probably guess why!

In the meantime, many of us still love to eat meat. However, to be on the safe side it would be advisable to eat a little less of it in the future. As meat and cheese are the main offenders in disrupting our sleeping patterns, these foods are probably better avoided. Drinking herbal teas and paying attention to the food we eat will help to avoid the cycle of sleeping tablets. As a result, we will feel healthier and fitter after a good night's natural sleep.

CHAPTER SEVEN

ALLERGIES

I have written extensively on the subject of allergies in my book *Viruses, Allergies and the Immune System*. An increasing number of people are experiencing allergy problems and it is quite sad to see that the allergic response is often taken out of context.

We have to realise that when one becomes allergic the immune system is often depressed, and that there are many causes that can trigger allergic reactions. Some simple allergy tests will reveal the causes and it is very often interesting to see how allergies disappear when the avoidance or elimination of certain foods is introduced.

Formerly, infections were the most frequent causes of disease. In our time allergies, mainly from food, are increasing uncontrollably. Over 70 per cent of the population of the industrial countries have an allergic disposition. Allergies are 'new' diseases which in the past were hardly known. When speaking of an allergy, we mean a *changed or unusual defensive reaction against specific well-known, or unknown, substances*. An allergic disposition can be hereditary or acquired. An allergic reaction to a substance or to food can occur within seconds, or over a period of up to 72 hours. Innumerable health problems and even serious illness can be caused by allergens. Most affected are the skin and the mucus membranes. There is no need to describe here the very complicated process which can trigger off an allergic reaction; this theme has often been described elsewhere. However, what we want to know is *why* we become allergic.

Until about 100 years ago an allergy was something out of the ordinary. Now it is officially accepted that the contamination of our modern environment has created a climate propitious for the development of such illnesses. We can get an allergy at any time in life, even as a bottle-fed baby. The organism of the baby has been intended for the digestion of mother's milk, which has a completely different quality and composition from cow's milk. A baby cannot completely assimilate and digest cow's milk or any other milk from animals, even if this has been changed in many ways in order to resemble human milk. In such milk there are always some foreign substances which cannot be digested or eliminated, and the organism of the baby must somehow get rid of these, as they interfere with many internal procedures. The easiest way for the organism to excrete these substances is through the skin and in this case the baby will get all kinds of skin problems, for example 'milk crust', from which many babies suffer. If these skin problems are not treated correctly, or the symptoms are suppressed by medication, very often more serious diseases may develop and the baby will retain an allergic disposition throughout its entire life. Such a baby will develop a great sensitivity to all kinds of allergens (substances which trigger an allergic reaction in the body), not only to those from milk and milk products.

More and more people are becoming allergic to milk and dairy products. Different kinds of cereals, especially wheat, refined carbohydrates, eggs, citrus fruits (mainly when they have been sprayed or waxed), tomatoes, chocolate, sausages, pork, breakfast cereals and tinned food can also cause allergic reactions.

At the beginning of the twentieth century there were only a few food additives on the market; nowadays there are thousands of them, as well as innumerable foreign substances from the environment. It is logical that the human organism tries to defend itself against all these toxins. Even when a certain substance is harmless in itself, it is possible that through its combination with other additives new and often very toxic substances can come into being. In medicine these dangers are known and many books have been written on the subject, but in the food industry they are completely ignored.

PHOSPHATES IN FOOD

Some of the food additives used most frequently today are phosphates, which are considered harmless by the official authorities, provided that their daily intake is no more than 750mg per day. Phosphates really can do miracles. By using these, dull, unattractive, old and wilted food can be made to look fresh and appetising once more. (Do you remember what I wrote with reference to the fodder of animals?) These phosphates are used in the cheese and meat industry, and in manufacturing cakes, pastries, soups, sauces, chocolate, soft drinks etc. They have excellent qualities as buffers, emulsifiers, thickening agents, coagulators and water absorbents, and for rendering certain substances inactive.

The foods which children like best are embellished and improved by phosphates in order to make them more attractive. Sausages, hamburgers, soft drinks, ice cream, pastries, sweets, puddings, and so on – everything contains phosphates. Therefore children often consume more than twice the amount recommended for adults.

Symptoms from an overdose of phosphates are often quite serious. One of these is MCD, minimal cerebral dysfunction. Other symptoms are hyper-activity, hypo-activity and autism. Hyperactive children fidget all the time and never keep quiet. Hypoactive and autistic children, on the contrary, have lost all *joie de vivre* and seem to have no energy at all.

ANTISOCIAL BEHAVIOUR

Disturbed muscular functions and uncontrolled movements.

Congenital alexia: children with spelling and reading problems.

Lack of concentration, children cannot listen.

Fear of physical contact.

Osteoporosis, disorders of bone-healing.

Pylorus cramps; cramps of the stomach muscles.

Pseudo croup, coughing fits because of restricted air-passage.

Disorders of the heart muscle.

Allergies: asthma, hay fever, nettle rash, eczema.

Different skin diseases, e.g. neurodermatitis.

Vasomotoric disorders, e.g. migraine.

Disorders of the stomach and intestinal dysfunctions.

Ulcers of the stomach or ulcers of the duodenum.

Herta Hafer, the author of the book *The Secret Drug: Food Phosphates*, gives the reader many sound arguments and proofs of the dangers of phosphates. On this subject there has been much scientific research done, but for several reasons most of this has not been published or just simply ignored. Certainly, not all of the symptoms mentioned above come only from an overdose of phosphates, and every disease has more than one cause, but it is high time to research the situation more thoroughly. Not only children but also adults become ill and suffer because of the irresponsible attitude of manufacturers!

Not only industrial products, but also natural products can contain allergens from agriculture or cattle breeding. One can react allergically to almost anything and such a reaction can take place in every part of the body. An allergic disposition can be dormant for many years and break out only after the person in question comes into contact with certain allergens while his defensive forces are under par.

Headaches, dizziness or migraine headaches that occur more or less regularly can be the first signs of an allergy. People who are suffering from bronchitis, sinusitis or asthma often owe their disease to an allergic disposition. The same applies in the case of tachycardia (a rapid heart beat), shortage of breath and similar problems. If the cause of the allergy can be discovered and removed, it is often surprising how quickly many health problems will disappear. But most of the time it is very difficult to find these allergens.

An allergic reaction can be caused by an addiction to certain kinds of food. If, for example, a person loves to eat chocolate and eats this almost every day, certain defensive reactions against the very concentrated contents become overstrained. This reaction can be against refined sugar, industrial cocoa or saturated fats, and it becomes impossible for the organism to replace the specific defensive cells needed quickly enough. In this case the body has to take other measures and any part of the body will co-operate in order to defend itself against the allergens. This situation can be compared to an army: when some special troops are unable to continue to fight, other units have to take over. The next battle will then perhaps be fought somewhere else, with different weapons. The same happens in the human body and far more diseases than we generally believe are caused by allergens, that is by certain substances with which our body can no longer cope.

Unfortunately most doctors do not understand this and they treat, for example, any asthmatic reaction or bronchitis with medication which suppresses the symptoms. That the patient in question could be, for example, allergic to cow's milk, sugar, chocolate, beer or certain chemical substances in the food is completely ignored. Because of this, millions of patients have to take suppressive medication throughout their whole lives. Any patient with such chronic health problems should at least try to cut out of his diet, for one or two weeks, any food which he eats regularly. It is very possible that a health problem he or she has had for years will disappear completely when the offensive substance is taken away.

People who get allergic reactions after eating their favourite food should refrain from having it in the future. Allergic problems can also be traced by watching a change in behaviour patterns. Often it is not the food itself but the additives in the food which cause allergies. In that case it is easy to explain why people are not always allergic to the same food. If there are no additives in the food, there will be no allergic reactions.

CHAPTER EIGHT

Mental Diseases

I n early antiquity people believed that mental diseases were caused by the wrath of the gods; insane people or their ancestors had been afflicted with this wrath because of wrong behaviour, and for this they had to suffer. One avoided such people, locked them up, or pitied them.

Formerly, hardly anybody would have thought that mental diseases, psychical problems or unusual behaviour could have anything to do with food allergies. This changed when some doctors in North America, England and later in Germany started to look into these problems. People like Ted Randolph, Herbert Rinkel, Albert Rowe, George Watson, Professor Comrey, Richard Mackarness, Professor Pfister, Lothar Burgerstein, Anna Calantin and many others achieved outstanding results in this field.

It became known that Hippocrates (460 BC) and other famous doctors of antiquity treated people who were mentally ill with laxatives, emetics and special diets, with much success. They were convinced that mental diseases and abnormal behaviour were often caused by a malfunction of the metabolism and not by a sick mind or a bad or unbalanced personality.

Some of the physicians mentioned above proved, 50 years ago, that a criminal mind can often be linked to wrong nutritional habits and to some specific foods in particular. They discovered that many criminals lived almost exclusively on so-called junk food or fast food and ate fried chicken with French fries regularly, often cooked in the same old oil, which had been reheated many times. Old, rancid oil is not only a vitamin and mineral robber; it can also damage and paralyse brain or nerve cells. Many criminals often act like zombies, as if they are in a kind of trance and do not really know what is going on. It is interesting that some hyperactive children often behave in a similar way. Of course, the oil is not the only culprit, but in combination with other refined and unnatural foods, it will be harmful not only for the body, but also for the mind.

POSSIBLE CAUSES OF MENTAL PROBLEMS AND MENTAL ILLNESS

Insane people have been treated in different ways throughout the years, and most often the mind was the main object of the treatment. Sometimes they were treated with love and affection, but more often very drastic measures were applied. One of these was electric shock treatment, which even today is still practised from time to time.

The Treatment of Mental Diseases

Hippocrates and other physicians in antiquity were far ahead of their time; in the case of mental illness they always treated the whole person, body and mind. In our time, since Sigmund Freud and the beginning of psychotherapy, patients who are mentally ill and people who suffer from depression, extreme mood swings, fear, restlessness, nervousness, aggressiveness etc. are mainly treated with psychological drugs and psychotherapy. Electric shock and similar treatments are rare. Modern medicine, by using drugs, has made much progress in treating mental illness. As the need arises, tranquillisers or stimulants are used; these are very successful in suppressing the symptoms. Now, many schizophrenic patients can stay at home; they receive outpatient treatment and can live a normal life. Hats off to the chemical industry!

However, all is not as good as it seems to be. Most of these drugs have not only physical but also very serious psychological side-effects. They paralyse certain nerve centres in the brain, and patients who take tranquillisers regularly often live permanently in a daze. They feel like zombies and cannot enjoy life anymore. Patients who are given stimulants, on the other hand, live in a state of permanent euphoria. This is extremely tiring, uses up all their available energy and can disturb normal body functions.

'New' Diseases

Although mental hospitals temporarily are no longer filled up, Alzheimer's patients or patients with similar diseases now take up all the vacant space. As the causes of these diseases still seem to be unknown, medicine can only treat the symptoms with special drugs. Obviously physicians do not know what else they can do, and to suggest completely different ways of treatment would be regarded as heretical.

During the last 50–100 years neurotic and psychosomatic diseases have increased enormously. At the same time the production of artificial and processed food, which is unsuitable for the human organism but is a wonderful money-maker, has greatly increased. When people consume this kind of food, not only the body but also the brain and the nervous system are bound to become ill. In addition, there is the rapidly increasing contamination of the environment in the industrial countries by electro-magnetic radiation. There is a strong possibility that such radiation has a great influence on the general state of our health and on our brain and nervous system.

Unfortunately, it is impossible to write in greater detail about this very interesting subject within the framework of this book.

METABOLIC DISORDERS AND MENTAL ILLNESS

There are still many scientists and physicians who do not believe that our metabolism could have anything to do with mental disorders. However, many years ago Sigmund Freud was already thinking about just such a possibility.

Anyone who has studied Freud's original publications knows that this great scientist was convinced that some day medicine would find an organic cause for most mental disorders. The physicians from North America and Europe mentioned earlier were very successful in finding absolute proof of Freud's theory.

> Every physician who takes the trouble to read something about the connections there are between mental diseases and nutrition could obtain surprising results by treating their patients while using this knowledge. (From *Not All in the Mind* by Richard Mackarness.)

DEPRESSION AND MOOD SWINGS

We all know that low blood sugar, for example, can cause fatigue and depression. As soon as the blood sugar is again normal, the depression disappears and the person in question feels relaxed. When one suffers from constipation, one very likely gets a headache or other complaint. With every metabolic problem one feels unwell, physically as well as mentally. Many people do not realise this and, instead of changing first their unhealthy eating and living habits, they go to a psychiatrist. In North America this has even become a fashionable habit; for any real or imaginary mental problem many people consult their 'shrink' regularly, often several times a week. Such treatment is expensive and is not always successful.

Body and mind should be seen as an integral whole, and treating depression and mental problems using only a one-sided psychological treatment makes no sense. Metabolic disorders should be diagnosed and treated as well. People who often suffer from depression or mood swings – up one minute, down the next – should look critically at their daily menu and living habits. Sometimes the person in question subconsciously knows exactly what he or she is doing wrong.

Such problems are often at least partly due to nutritional disorders or food allergies. A lack of fresh air, exercise and enough sleep also play an important role in the case of these problems. At the same time there can be a lack of vitamins and minerals and additives, drugs, insecticides, fertilisers and other chemical substances may be responsible for these health problems.

If the liver or kidney function is impaired, these organs will be unable to neutralise and eliminate enough toxins. As a consequence of internal infections the organism sometimes produces too many metabolic toxins. Many medicaments have side-effects, some of which are mental.

CHANGE OF DIET AND VITAMINS

Many years ago a well-known German physician wrote: 'How much misery, how many mistakes, how many frictions are nothing else but the effects of metabolic toxins on the human personality.' Max Bircher-Benner, too, knew about the constant interactions of the mind and the body. Very early he realised that a one-sided treatment of any disease is never sufficient.

On a biochemical level, there is always more proof of a very close link between the intake and assimilation of different nutrients and mental health. In the case of depression there is often a lack of vitamins B or C;

magnesium and calcium help one relax; pantothenic acid, one of the B vitamins, relieves tension and provides sound sleep; and a lack of niacin (vitamin B3) or folic acid can trigger off depression, tiredness and fatigue. Other symptoms are often caused by a lack of chromium.

A list of such symptoms of deficiency could be quite a long one. However, one should always realise that most vitamins nowadays are produced synthetically and can never replace the natural nutrients one finds in healthy food. Although such vitamins and minerals can solve the worst problems temporarily, usually a change of diet is needed in order to become really healthy.

The bacterial flora in the intestines should be treated with natural remedies and the bowel movement should be normalised. When all the body functions have again become normal, most mental problems usually disappear as well. Problems that seemed to be insurmountable do not appear so bad anymore. A healthy body can handle stress and mental problems much better than a body which is weak and ill.

When patients eventually realise that their physical and mental health lie in their own hands and are their own responsibility, diseases that seemed to be incurable often disappear in a very short time.

The many mental, cerebral and nervous diseases which are now increasing in a frightening way should, and could, be treated differently. In any case, one can always at least try to resort to some of the methods of treatment described in the three volumes of this book. Physicians who would be open-minded enough to try this could be very successful.

Anita Backhaus, the author of the book *Healing Without*

Medication or Injections, in which she relates her experiences in her water clinic in Colombia, says:

> I am completely convinced that mental stress is caused mainly by different infections in the intestines. Those could be cured by fasting, a change of diet, natural remedies and the application of several intestinal baths, whereby enemas with up to 40 litres of water are used for cleaning out the bowels and the intestines.
>
> In 90 per cent of all cases of mental problems, the intestines are weak and do not function properly and such a treatment would show surprising results. In that case the physician does not have to rack his brains about the patient's emotional problems, as the real cause lies in a constantly toxically contaminated organism.

She is 100 per cent correct in what she says!

CHAPTER NINE

Mental Attitude

Throughout this book, in which we have discussed the ten golden rules for healthy living, we have mainly concentrated on food, rest and relaxation – in other words, the main influencing factors in our daily lives. Today's society and the current hectic pace of life has disrupted our natural behaviour patterns. Personally, I stipulate to every patient that it is not difficult to live life as our body requires. It is not mathematics; by considering our circumstances sensibly and realistically we can easily make the necessary adjustments to become both healthier and happier.

Food is certainly a major influence. I am also aware that there are addictions that cannot be easily overcome. Our attitude has to be positive in overcoming any problem. We should not say to ourselves, 'I cannot do this', or 'This is too difficult'. Be positive! I can understand that once you have read through this book, it may seem that everything we like to eat is forbidden and unhealthy. It is likely that you may be asking yourself, 'What am I allowed to eat?'

Mainly for this reason, and because there are so many different opinions about what is healthy or unhealthy, most people do not even begin changing their eating habits. While one is still young and more or less healthy, this does not seem to be very important. However, by the time one gets older, not so healthy anymore, or even suffering from some chronic disease, things are different.

As more then 70 per cent, or according to some people more then 90 per cent, of all civilisation diseases are caused by our modern nutrition, even the best doctor cannot cure such a disease if the patient does not change his or her nutritional habits. Healthy food can be varied and very tasty, and can be adjusted to all personal likes and dislikes. But changing your eating habits should not be done all of a sudden. Many patients who understand that this is their last chance to get well change their eating habits quite suddenly and this is wrong. After only a few days, these people will get a stomach- ache and other complaints and will convince themselves that this 'healthy food' does not agree with them. They are discouraged and will not make the effort to eat differently. They will eat the same kind of food as they ate before and their disease will become worse. If, however, the change of diet is done in the right way, there will already be after some weeks or even days a positive change in the state of the patient's health. This becomes a real challenge and when the symptoms go away the person in question will be delighted. While changing the diet, the individual's reactions to different kinds of food should always be taken into consideration and the changes should be made step by step. To take it easy is the best way.

How to do it

1. First of all you should eliminate from your menu all foods which generally do most harm; these are denatured and industrialised foods.

You should eat less and less refined sugar, flour and refined fats, or foods containing these products. If this is difficult for you, you can use in the beginning some honey, pure maple syrup or something similar. Stevia is a new, completely natural sweetener from the juice of a plant, which was used in olden times by the Indians.

For some people a change of diet will be more difficult than for others, especially for those who were used to eating many sweets and desserts. However, it is interesting that after eating only natural sweets like honey or sweet fruits, after some time the craving for sugar disappears.

2. If you are used to eating big helpings and to eating between meals often, you will now have to get used to eating only one or two meals, and half the quantity you are used to. This is not difficult to learn if each time you take a smaller portion and chew each bite for a longer time. In the beginning you may be hungry between meals, and you may get tired sooner. In that case you can eat (slowly!) one or two pieces of fruit mid-morning or mid-afternoon, or if this does not help, once in a while you can eat instead of fruit a small portion of boiled unsweetened oats.

Of course, you will still make many mistakes, especially in the beginning, and you will probably be easily tempted to eat something unhealthy. However, after some time you will get used to the new way of eating. Surprisingly, sweets will not taste as good as before and after eating something that is not so healthy you will find you do not feel so good. Usually there will be a great improvement in health, and people again begin to enjoy life.

3. When after some weeks you have become used to eating healthier food, you can take the next step on the road to health. From now on one should really eat more, though at the most three times a day without any snacks, the only exception being some fruit. In this manner the digestive system can take a rest between meals.

For breakfast you can either eat fruit, a well-prepared muesli or some wholewheat bread with a little butter and honey, or you can enjoy a hearty spread from the health food shop. With breakfast you can drink herb tea or decaffeinated coffee with a little cream, but no sugar.

At midday, you may start with a little bowl of salad, with the right kind of salad dressing (some cold-pressed oil, a little lemon juice or apple vinegar, some sea or herbal salt, and herbs). After the salad you can eat two or three different vegetables; the best way is to steam them, and jacket potatoes or whole rice, polenta or another cereal dish. Never use any kind of fat or oil when you prepare these foods. However, when they are on your plate you can add a little butter or cold-pressed vegetable oil. You can eat meat, fish or eggs in the beginning, about two or three times a week, but later you should eat less of these.

With the exception of soybeans or bean sprouts, I do not recommend that you eat too many soya or similar products. As you have read, all foods when they are processed lose with each step much of their original value. Soya and similar products are intensively processed and after all these treatments they could not possible contain many ingredients which are valuable for our health. Everyone can understand this. Wholemeal cereals are far healthier than all these new and foreign products of which even the biological origin is never quite certain.

Always, especially in the beginning, your meals should be as simple as possible. A vegetable or cereal dish, a cereal soup, muesli or something similar will do. If, at the beginning, you still want to drink coffee or black tea it does not matter. However, if your disease is serious and you want to get completely well, you should follow all the advice given in this book.

Although a change of diet is extremely important, this diet therapy should, especially in the case of serious and chronic diseases, be supported by natural healing methods and remedies.

ADDICTION AS THE CAUSE OF ILLNESS

Many people are addicted in one way or another. Some don't even know that they are addicted. They are convinced that only chain-smokers, for example, are addicts.

There are various forms of addiction: there is addiction to bread, chocolate, ice cream, coffee, alcohol, drugs, sweets or cola drinks. There is gluttony, anorexia, obesity, bulimia etc. Some addictions are more dangerous than others, but no addiction is harmless. Some addictions which are related to nutrition can be caused by a malfunction of the pancreas, but all addictions have the same origin. Addicted people yearn for something they miss or lack, not only emotionally but also physically. For instance, why does a person become an alcoholic? Some people who have a personal problem start drinking to calm down. Emotional problems give the first incentive towards addiction and many doctors still believe that physiological problems and too little willpower are the only causes of addiction.

That addictive behaviour can also have physical causes is hardly known. Although some people may drink once, twice or three times too much if they have a personal problem, only a small percentage of these people really become addicted to alcohol. Why does one person become an alcoholic and another person not? It is certainly not a question of character. The problem lies elsewhere.

The need for certain nutrients is different with every person. There are people who need a lot more of some vitamins, minerals or vital substances than others. Many people, even if they eat healthy food, often cannot assimilate or store these vital nutrients. In order to assimilate and process alcohol, coffee, sweets or, even in the case of non-smokers, cigarette smoke, the organism uses up great amounts of vital nutrients.

When a person who leads a healthy life (if that is still possible in this day and age) drinks a little too much from time to time, it won't harm them. However, if somebody else who suffers from a chronic lack of vital nutrients does the same, he/she will become an alcoholic sooner or later, depending on his/her state of health. With every glass of wine or cigarette, a greater desire develops which cannot be met in the long run. The person concerned feels that he/she lacks something and becomes nervous and restless. Then he/she will again reach for the glass, a cigarette or the drugs, and the vicious circle continues. In this way the person in question gets deeper and deeper into the addiction.

Many of these people have been convinced by their physician or by their friends that their addiction only comes from their weak character. Because of this they often go into deep depression, and over and over again they succumb to their addiction. It is hardly possible for them to get out of this vicious circle by themselves. One cannot do it alone.

THESE PEOPLE NEED HELP – BUT HOW?

The most important thing is that the person in question really wants to get rid of his addiction. If the addiction has already become stronger than the desire for health, there is no need for the addict to bother at all – he/she no longer cares. Some people have found help with AA (Alcoholics Anonymous). If one becomes a member of this charitable organisation one is no longer allowed to drink a single drop of alcohol. This is very difficult for most alcoholics and only a few can keep it up. There is always the possibility of a relapse, even after many years. But this international organisation has achieved a lot of success and continues to do so. It should be viewed with great respect. If they go into a clinic for detoxification, alcoholics are practically locked up for weeks and sometimes for months. Nobody there is allowed to drink alcohol and the common treatment consists of psychotherapy and pharmaceutical drugs, which often increase the lack of vital nutrients! After such a detoxification treatment and recovery there are often relapses. AA, and most hospitals, try to influence the addicted person's personality and behaviour. They want to change a weak character and strengthen the willpower. If people believe in God or another superior power, one tries to influence their wish to be abstinent through religious thoughts and prayers. Sometimes this works and people don't suffer a relapse.

Life is very hard for such ex-alcoholics; often they do not enjoy life anymore because they live in fear of their own weakness. It is unbelievable how much distress and misery such a one-sided therapy can cause.

However, for many years well-informed doctors and naturopaths have known that there are also other reasons for an addiction. An addiction can be caused by:

◆ an abnormal need of certain vital nutrients (e.g. B vitamins)
◆ food allergies
◆ nutrition which lacks many vital substances
◆ food additives and junk food
◆ too many refined carbohydrates
◆ a weak immune system
◆ an environment containing many toxins
◆ great worries, anxiety and other personal problems

Most often a combination of the various causes mentioned above triggers an addiction. Therefore it is important to have certain tests done. Among these are hair, blood and blood sugar tests, which should be done regularly in order to find out which deficiencies, allergies, toxic or poisonous substances are involved. With the help of these tests it will be possible to compose a very personal diet for the patients and to supply them with the nutrients they lack. Every person who suffers from addiction should be treated in the same way as people who suffer from other diseases. The organism should first be cleaned and the further intake of harmful substances should be strictly avoided. Fasting is very important. And one should get into the habit of always eating as healthily as possible. Bowel movements should be regular and the bacterial flora should be sanitised. The intestines should be cleansed by enemas with chamomile tea and sometimes colon hydrotherapy can do miracles. Sufficient physical exercise and fresh air are very important.

The worst problem for the patient is total abstinence. To drink a glass of wine, not every day but now and then, can be very enjoyable. Even in ancient times, people liked to have a drink in order to relax. Yet this treat was always reserved for exceptional festive occasions. Providing the patient is not yet too addicted, total abstinence will only be necessary for a certain time, i.e. until there is no more lack of various vital substances, which can be proved by different tests. After this, he/she will be allowed to drink one to two glasses of wine occasionally, e.g. when there is a family party, but especially in the beginning his/her drinking habits will have to be strictly watched. Usually there will be no relapse if the person concerned always remembers to take a mixture of the substances he/she lacks. There are specific nutrients which all alcoholics lack, and other substances would have to be tailored to the needs of each patient individually.

As long as our 'civilisation food' is deficient in many ways, addictions will increase and the general health of the population will worsen.

The treatment mentioned above is the only one which might really at last help some addicted persons and their relatives. Unfortunately, many doctors and nurses, and people with stubborn and dogmatic attitudes, will continue to ignore the facts mentioned above. It will be very difficult to change this kind of attitude as there is much ignorance, but eventually common sense may again conquer dogmatism. Then millions of people could be helped in a much better and more sensible way.

What causes illness in our time?

In our time illness is caused mainly by toxins, poisons, unusable residues and many substances produced by a diseased environment. To make it easier for the reader we will simply call all of these substances 'toxins'. All toxins should be dissolved, broken up and moved to the execrative organs, where they can be disposed of.

Toxins are substances which get into our body by way of food and through the respiratory tract and the skin; they also develop in our body, coming from metabolic waste, morbid cells, dead bacteria, residues of cells etc. These toxins are, as the famous 'water doctor' Priessnitz, used to say: 'All substances that cannot be assimilated and become part of the fundamental substances of our body.'

Harmful toxins are, among others:

◆ 2,500 officially registered food additives
◆ chemical residues from agriculture, like fertilisers, insecticides, herbicides, etc.
◆ chemical and synthetic drugs
◆ harmful gases, like tobacco smoke, exhaust fumes, paint, different sprays, etc.

◆ deodorants, vaginal sprays, perfume, cosmetics, washing and cleaning substances, soap, etc.

Such toxins, which are foreign substances for our organism and have no business being there, get into the body by way of the intestines, the lungs, the skin and the mucus membranes, eventually accumulating in all body tissues. They can also damage our vital organs and, as for our organism, it is no natural task to deal with such foreign matter – our defensive mechanisms are constantly overtaxed. Many of these toxins originate in the organism itself, especially from the polluted contents of our intestines.

Presently, medicine does not understand that all our 'new diseases' have a completely different origin to the former infectious diseases. It is very careless and irresponsible to treat such completely different diseases in exactly the same manner as infections would be treated. Hippocrates said: 'The first law while treating a patient is "never to do any harm".' However, a host of physicians, often without realising it, offend almost daily against this law! It is sad when these mistakes are made.

One's mental attitude should be positive. Daily I come across people who are reluctant to give up certain foods or do not wish to give up smoking or drinking. When I give these people acupuncture treatment, I ask them to mentally repeat 'I want to'. To repeatedly think, 'I want to be healthy. I want to be well and I can do it!' can bring about amazing results and changes. You should believe in yourself before you become ill and it is too late.

I have often seen patients lose the battle because they continue to delay making the necessary changes. Be positive in your attitude. You can do it! There is enough willpower in all of us; if you want to do something, you will achieve your goal. I look at the hundreds of letters that I have received from people who were in dire straits. They have turned their lives around and are now so much happier and healthier. The changes have all been worth it!

The ten simple golden rules are easy to follow. Make the changes in your mind and start today, not tomorrow!

CHAPTER TEN

Visualisation

As we approach the end of the book, we come to what is perhaps the best golden rule – visualisation. I often say in my lectures that the mind is stronger than the body and it is well known that creative visualisation can be of invaluable help. In simple terms, this involves creating a picture in one's mind of a situation or an event that you wish to occur. By enforcing this message to the brain, and the brain accepting the picture as a command, you are able to turn visualisation into reality. Realism does not always come into it. Simply visualising the way or manner you wish a situation to develop or progress can have surprising effects. I have often been amazed over the years at how effective visualisation can be. The mind is indeed stronger than the body.

Happiness can be achieved by visualising that you *are* the type of happy person you wish to be. Creative visualisation is done on a daily basis. It is not only meditation but visualisation that can help you to become a happy and healthy person, rather than one who moans and groans on Monday morning. Instead of doing this, take some time out to visualise and do some of the exercises that I will discuss to help your mind tune into the things that you desire to happen.

Creative visualisation can also be of great help in an emergency, or in an urgent situation. Concentrating one's mind on visualising a desirable outcome, especially when things appear to have a poor outlook, is a very wise thing to do. This is what Dr Carl Simonton, a radiologist and oncologist, and his wife Natalie Simonton, a psychotherapist, noticed with their patients. In dealing with his patients, Dr Simonton clearly saw what visualisation could and did achieve, and demonstrated this by employing several methods, one or two of which I will describe later in this chapter. In general, patients often negatively view their particular situation or problem as so bad that they think it will never get better or, as I often hear, they exclaim: 'I have got a problem and I really can't live with it any longer.' The Simontons clearly saw that this is not just purely a physical problem, but a problem that also affects the person's mental and emotional well-being.

It is possible to strengthen the immune system by way of relaxation and visualisation techniques. In following these methods, the Simontons had great success with their patients and even when dealing with the most difficult of their patients' problems, they drew comfort from knowing that the visualisation techniques would be of benefit.

Nature is remarkable in that millions of repair cells are available for our bodies to utilise. These repair cells appear to be intelligent and responsive to our thoughts: if we influence our cells positively towards any healing process, an enormous army of cells sets to work to heal the body with the great power that God has bestowed on us. Responding to even minor vibrations, our body cells possess an innate intelligence enabling them to follow our directions. If we therefore look at perfect images and are imaginative in rebuilding the creative energy, a higher level of improvement can be achieved. These vibrations can be thoughts or actions and will result in reactions. Perhaps we can now understand how a positive mental and emotional attitude can readily help us to a manifestation of good health and strength. We can then also understand that the healing of disease by such positive elements of love and happiness will be victorious over emotions like fear, worry, hate, anxiety, envy, stress or any other destructive vibrations.

Since I began to instruct patients in visualisation or relaxation techniques, I have seen many cases which proved their effectiveness. After years of experience, I am strongly of the opinion that cancer can be overcome, as well as possibly prevented, by establishing the right positive attitudes and vibrations within the body. Sometimes a misconception needs to be cleared away first. I recall a lady who once asked me, 'How can a dead cell come back to life once it's dead?' I had to inform her that once a cell has died, it will remain dead because it cannot be reanimated. Even God will not bring a dead cell back to life. Yet a dead cell or a carcinomic cell can be disposed of and replaced by a new cell. Let us consider that every six months in an adult life the cells are replaced. If a cell stays in the body for longer than this it can more readily become a carcinomic cell. So we come back to the importance of dietary management. It is to our advantage to use the life force within the food we eat for the renewal of cells. It is unfortunate that generally people are unwilling to change their eating habits unless they become aware of medical complications. Often common sense does not prevail till then. It seems to present less of a problem for people to change their religion, their political views, or their husband or wife! I have seen how difficult it is for most to change their eating habits.

A change in dietary management is unlikely to produce immediate results. After all, the problem did not spring up overnight. Be optimistic and never give in by saying, 'I am going to die' or 'I will never get better'. Instead reprogramme the mind with 'I am basically healthy and therefore I will be victorious over my problems'. Always remember that without our life force we are lost.

The old naturopathic views on the beneficial effects of sunshine, fresh air and exercise are thankfully back in focus today. Healthy breathing will indeed help the vital processes in the body which depend on oxygen. Take exercise in the fresh air whenever possible as this is always advantageous.

Do not be easily discouraged, because it is essential to understand that we have to be wholehearted in our efforts. The heart is the only organ that can never be attacked by cancer. Let us meditate on the thought that if our heart is full of love, how much love we will then receive as a healing factor. This is the meaning of the visualisation or autogenic techniques, or any other positive attitude techniques that will help us to overcome our troubles.

I would like to end this book with a few guidelines for some of these simple techniques, although there are dozens of examples that can easily be obtained from a variety of organisations or books on the subject.

The first of these is a very worthwhile bone-breathing visualisation exercise. The Chinese believe that the centre of your bones is responsible for the well-being of the body as a whole. This exercise in visualisation, together with the relaxation that goes with it, is widely used as a therapy for those with bone disorders.

You will use your breath by imagining the breath entering up and through the bones as you breathe in and, and as you breathe out, being passed down and away through the same path.

The first thing is to get yourself into a comfortable position, either in a sitting position, in a comfortable upright chair, feet placed evenly on the floor, hands resting in the lap, spine straight and the head resting comfortably, with the top of the head in line with the ceiling, or lying down on a comfortable mat with the spine straight, arms to the side with the palms turned upwards, feet just a little way apart.

Begin to become aware of your breathing. Slow the breath right down, making it as slow and deep as you can. Feel the breath right down to the bottom of the ribcage as you breathe in deep, slow, even breaths. Begin to feel the body relaxing as you concentrate your mind on the breath coming in and out, relaxing and letting go.

Now begin the visualisation:

◆ Imagine the breath coming into and through the bones of the left foot, up the bones of the leg to the hip bone. Then, as you breathe out, the breath returns the same way and out through the left foot. Repeat seven times.

◆ Imagine the breath coming in and up through the

bones of the right foot, up the bones of the leg to the hip and then, as you breathe out, imagine the breath returning the same way and out through the right foot. Repeat seven times.

◆ Breathe in through the bones of the left foot up the left leg, cross through the pelvis and, as you breathe out, send the breath down the bones and out through the right foot. Repeat seven times.

◆ Breathe in and up through the bones of the left hand, up through the bones of the left arm to the shoulder. Breathe out and return down and out the same way. Repeat seven times.

◆ Breathe in and up through the bones of the right hand and up the right arm, to the shoulder. Then breathe out and down the same way. Repeat seven times.

◆ Breathe in through the left arm and across from the left shoulder to the right shoulder, then breathe out down the right arm and through the bones of the right hand. Breathe in and up to the left shoulder and breathe out down the left arm and out through the left hand. Repeat seven times.

◆ Breathing in, take the breath up the spine to the top, and then, as you breathe out, send the breath down the spine again and out through the base. Repeat seven times.

◆ Imagine the skull. Take a breath in and direct it up and over the head to the front, breathing out. Take the breath out through the skull and back. Repeat seven times.

◆ Now imagine the body as a whole. Take the breath in, up from both feet and up through all the bones

in the body to the top of the head, breathing down
and out through all the bones and out through the
feet. Repeat seven times.

It may be easier to visualise the breath in terms of a colour,
a light or a feeling of warmth, whatever you find the
easiest, and repeat the whole exercise as often as you like.
It may seem a little difficult at first, especially if this is the
first time you have done any visualisation, but persevere
and soon it will flow and you will receive great benefit.

Sometimes people practise something between
relaxation and visualisation, and also between visualisation
and taking back their strength. And that is going, in your
mind, to a place you like very much. See yourself in a
beautiful park, under a particularly lovely tree, or
somewhere in the mountains, or perhaps at the side of a
lake. Just choose a place you like very much and study
everything around you. Hear the birds, breathe the fresh
air, feel and smell the grass. Make all your senses
participate in this exercise. It is a good preparation for the
visualisation.

Do the bone-breathing exercise three times daily. Make
sure you cannot be interrupted during this period. Take
fifteen to twenty minutes each time, because the steady
drop hollows the stone!

Do something about it today. Bear in mind the old
Sanskrit saying: 'Yesterday is but a dream, tomorrow is but
a vision. But today well-lived makes every yesterday a
dream of happiness and every tomorrow a vision of hope.
Look well therefore to this day.'

İndex